The Street-wise Popular Practical Guides

"Dr. Lefever has lived his life fighting his own demons and, having learned those lessons, helping tens of thousands of people to overcome theirs. No one has ever written better about addiction, with more insight, with more understanding, or with more compassion. Think of this book as the first step towards keeping families together."
– **Jeffrey Robinson**, best-selling author of *The Laundrymen*, etc.

"Unique insights into addictiveness. This guide is full of Robert Lefever's own experiences and personal wisdom peppered with stories of his patients both in and out of recovery. It will help many to make sense of their self-destructive behaviours and regain hope. Robert's maverick style belies the extraordinary transformation he has catalysed in many hundreds of lives as well as the scores of therapists he has trained and encouraged to join a much needed work force.
– **Dr. Michael Gormley**, FRCP.

'Wise and compassionate.
– **Stephen Pollard,** Editor, *The Jewish Chronicle.*

"For over thirty years I – and many others – have struggled to find the right words to explain addicts, addiction and recovery to those who do not inhabit our world. With compassion and humility, but also with clarity, Robert Lefever describes what is often frightening, distressing and bewildering for families and friends, but also for most healthcare professionals: the seemingly endless nightmare that is active addiction, and the mystery, both simple and at the same time complex, that is recovery from addiction.
"Lefever calls his book the Street-wise guide, and there are two streets where this book should be compulsory reading: Harley Street and Whitehall. There is everything in this book for the families and friends of addicts, to help them understand what is happening to the addict in their life, But it is perhaps even more important that the professionals to whom addicts and their families turn for help, and who often struggle to make sense of addiction, learn from a colleague who uses both his personal and professional experience to explain the theory and the practice of steering addicts from active addiction into a recovery that is both healthy and fulfilling. For the policy makers of Whitehall the lessons within Lefever's book could lead to a revolution in government's response to drug, alcohol, food and gambling addiction whether by the Department of Health or the Home Office.
– **Lord Benjamin Mancroft**.

The Street-wise Popular Practical Guides

The Street-wise Guide to Coping with and Recovering from Addiction

Robert Lefever

EER

Edward Everett Root, Publishers, Brighton, 2018.

EER

Edward Everett Root, Publishers, Co. Ltd.,
30 New Road, Brighton, Sussex, BN1 1BN, England.
www.eerpublishing.com

edwardeverettroot@yahoo.co.uk

EER Street-wise Guides, no.2.

Robert Lefever

The Street-wise Guide to Coping with and Recovering from Addiction

First published in Great Britain in 2018.

ISBN: 978-1-912224-48-7 paperback.
ISBN: 978-1-912224-47-0 hardback.
ISBN: 978-1-912224-49-4 ebook.

Typeset in Book Antiqua

Designed by Pageset Limited, High Wycombe, Buckinghamshire.
Printed in Great Britain by Lightning Source UK, Milton Keynes.

The Street-wise Popular Practical Guides

Edited by Karol Sikora and John Spiers.

This original paperback series provides *practical,* expert, insider-knowledge.

Each book tells you what professionals know, but which is not often shared with the public at large.

The books provide vital insider guidance, including what some authorities would prefer you never to know.

The authors are all internationally acknowledged professional experts and skilled popular writers.

We will be pleased to receive suggestions for other titles.

AVAILABLE.

Robert Lefever, *The Street-wise Guide to Coping with and Recovering from Addiction.*

Karol Sikora, *The Street-wise Patient's Guide To Surviving Cancer. How to be an active, organised, informed, and welcomed patient.*

Lady Teviot, *The Street-wise Guide to Doing Your Family History.*

FORTHCOMING.

Tom Balchin, *The Street-wise Guide to Surviving a Stroke.*

Georgina Burnett, *The Street-wise Guide to Buying, Improving, and Selling Your Home.*

Eamonn Butler, *The Street-wise Guide to the British Economy.*

Sam Collins, *The Street-wise Guide to Choosing a Care Home.*

Stephen Davies, *The Street-wise Guide to the Devil and His Works.*

John Hammond and Sara Thornton, *The Street-wise Guide to Weather Watching: The Elements Shaping Our Lives.*

Raj Persaud and Peter Bruggen, *The Street-wise Guide to Getting the Best Mental Health Care. How to Survive the Mental Health System and Get Some Proper Help.*

Gill Steel, *The Street-wise Guide to Getting The Best From Your Lawyer.*

To my late wife, Meg, for working with me in our rehab.

And to my wife, Pat, for all she does in keeping me young and happy – as well as for her patient editing skills.

About the author

Dr. Robert Lefever is internationally recognised as one of the best-known doctors who has specialised in addiction. He trained in Corpus Christi College, Cambridge and at The Middlesex Hospital, London. He created the first NHS group medical practice in South Kensington and one of the first private diagnostic centres in London. Then he set up the first rehab in the world to treat all addictive behaviour, and the depression and damaged self-esteem that underlies it, without using medicines except for detox. He is a regular national media commentator and columnist.

In 23 years he has treated over 5,000 in-patients suffering from various forms of addictive behaviour. He has visited the USA over 30 times, attending key conferences and seeing rehabs. He has lectured throughout the rest of the world on addiction and recovery.

Today he does his counselling work on an out-patient basis in South Kensington in London. He uses all his previous experience in focussing his attention, and confidential concern, on the patient sitting with him.

He and his wife, Pat, get to so many operas they wonder how they find time for their writing.

Contents

Contents

Key Terminology (my definitions)

Abuse:
A hurtful action in the perception of the recipient and maybe also in the view of others.

Addict:
Someone who cannot predict the extent of further compulsive behaviour after the first use of a mood-altering substance or process in any day.

Addiction:
A disorder of neurotransmission (the way one cell communicates with another) in the mood centres of the brain.

Addictive:
Something or somebody possessing a mood-altering effect.

Addictive behaviour:
Actions motivated by a desire to change the mood – wanting something out there to fix a sense of emptiness in here – regardless of damaging consequences.

Addictive characteristics:
Specific features of compulsive behaviour.

Addictive nature:
The (probably genetically determined) drive to change the mood regardless of circumstance.

Addictive outlet:
A substance, process or relationship that has a significant mood-altering effect on a particular individual.

Alcoholic:
Someone who uses alcohol primarily as a friend and comforter.

Allopathic:
Classically trained approaches to medication and therapy.

Alternative:
Therapeutic approaches that are generally outside the realm of standard medical practice.

Anonymous Fellowships:	Groups formed for mutual help through using the Twelve Step programme first formulated by Alcoholics Anonymous.
Big Book:	The familiar term for the book *Alcoholics Anonymous* that tells the story of how people surmount the ravages of dependency.
Blind Watchmaker:	Richard Dawkins' concept of evolution as opposed to creation.
CBT (Cognitive behavioural therapy):	A psychological process based on the belief that changes in thought will lead to change in behaviour.
Clinician:	Someone in the front line, rather than in the back room, when working with people to help them with their thoughts, feelings, behaviour and bodily function.
Codependency:	A term that means too many things – concerning the origins and current nature of particular relationships – to have any true consistent meaning. In my strict definition it means the mutual dance to death by an addict and a compulsive helper.
Compulsive behaviour:	Actions that escape comfortable control.
Compulsive helping:	Actions determined by the giver's need to be needed rather than by whether they actually help the recipient.
Counselling:	Talking therapies aimed at changing perceptions and behaviour.
Counsellors:	People who set themselves or up – sometimes with very little training or clinical experience – to be advisors on solving human problems.
Cravings:	The sense of inner compulsion to use a mood-altering substance, behaviour or relationship.

Detoxification:	Short-term use of medication and environmental support in order to help people to reduce dependency on mood-altering substances and processes.
Drug-dependent behaviour:	The state of being unable to live comfortably without using a mood-altering substance, behaviour or relationship.
Drug-seeking behaviour:	The preoccupation with finding a substance, behaviour or relationship to change the mood.
EMDR (Eye-Movement Desensitising and Reprocessing):	A therapeutic process that enables the 'thinking' brain to communicate with the 'feeling' brain.
Enabling:	Behaviour that permits and even overlooks the progressive and destructive addictive actions of someone else.
General Medical Council:	The UK doctors' disciplinary body that also regulates medical education.
Genetic predisposition:	Something determined by the way we are made rather than by our environment.
Harm minimisation:	The use of substitute drugs and sensible well-informed behaviour to counter addiction (although the most effective harm minimisation is, of course, abstinence).
Hazelden:	The first rehab in the world to treat addictive or compulsive behaviour (different terms for the same process) by using a combination of psychological approaches and the Twelve Step programme.
Hedonism:	The drive for pleasure irrespective of the damaging consequences to self or others. Ultimately, our addictive hedonism wants us dead.

Intervention: The structured process involved in confronting addictive behaviour in order to increase insight and lead to a willingness to accept help.

Memory blankouts: Loss of awareness of actions when under the influence of mood-altering substances, behaviours or relationships.

Metabolism: Body biochemistry and how it works.

Mood-altering behaviours: Actions and relationships that change the mood.

Mood-altering substances: Legal, illegal, prescribed or ingested substances that change the mood.

Mood centres: The parts of the brain that determine how we feel rather than how we act or perceive.

Neurotransmitters: Chemicals that transmit electrical impulses from one nerve ending to another.

NLP (Neuro-Linguistic Programming): The study and practice of the use of language in determining beliefs and behaviours.

Normies: An affectionate term used by addicts like me to describe people who have no addictive tendencies.

Osteoporosis: The crumbling of bones through defects in the metabolism of calcium.

People-pleasing: Emotionally driven actions that expect something in return from the recipient.

Physiological addiction: The temporary physical habituation that comes from repeated use.

Psychiatrist: A doctor who uses medication and challenges to thought processes in order to influence behaviour.

Psychodrama: A psychological process that uses action to interpret thoughts, feelings and behaviour in the past, and to influence them in the present or future.

Psychological techniques: Processes that are used therapeutically to influence behaviour.

Psychologist: A trained thinker and behaviourist who helps people to change thoughts, feelings and behaviour.

Psychopathology: A disorder of the mind negatively affecting perceptions and actions.

Psychotropic: A substance or behaviour that acts on the mind.

REBT (Rational Emotive Behaviour Therapy):   A psychological process that aims to enable people to talk back to inner voices and gain control over their behaviour.

Recovery: The state of peaceful acceptance and abstinence from use of mood-altering substances, behaviours and relationships as a result of daily working of the Twelve Step programme.

Recreational drugs: Non-prescribed substances that are used to alter the mood.

Rehab: An inpatient or outpatient facility that employs the Twelve Step programme alongside physical and psychological therapeutic processes in treating people with addiction problems.

Relapse: The process that begins with discontinuation of daily work on the Twelve Step programme and leads towards return to the addictive use of mood-altering substances, behaviours and relationships.

Self-esteem: The sense of self determined by our own actions.

Serenity: Peace of mind, acceptance and gratitude.

SMART Recovery: A psychological process that believes that inner resources are sufficient to tackle behavioural or external difficulties.

Spirituality: A sense of hope, trust, honour, innocence, peace, beauty, awareness and other abstract values that give meaning to life.

Therapeutic programme: A process that aims to help someone who has difficulty with thoughts, feelings and behaviour or with bodily processes.

Therapists and psychotherapists: People who generally charge more money than counsellors.

Twelve Step approach: Use of the Twelve Step programme, first formulated by Alcoholics Anonymous, in helping to counter addictive urges comfortably one day at a time.

Chapter 1: The Start

Addiction significantly affects 1 in 6 of us.

Addiction is an equal opportunity illness. It affects princes, paupers, politicians, professionals and people in general. Privilege gives no protection. Poverty is not a predictor.

Anyone can become physiologically addicted. Give someone a shot of morphine every day for a month and he or she will have withdrawal symptoms for a week or so if the drugs are stopped. But, for most people, once off there will be no craving to go back.

But some people – about one in six of the population – appear to have an addictive nature. Once starting to use a mood-altering substance in any day, there will often be a craving to continue. These people can give up for a time – a week, a month, a year or even more – but often become irritable. And at times they crave to return to former use.

They seem to have an in-born sense of inner emptiness. They discover for themselves that some substances and processes have a magical mood-altering effect. They ask themselves why they would ever stop using them. If life is grim, for one reason or another, and they feel down even at the best of times, it makes sense to them to use something that 'works'. Conversely, if at times they feel great and want to feel even greater, they see no earthly reason why not.

They discover that alcohol, nicotine, sugar, cannabis, cocaine and other substances 'work'. They hit the spot. So do gambling, work, exercise and various mood-altering behaviours. Potatoes and rhubarb do not work. Nor does learning about psychological techniques or getting involved in community activities.

For these people everything seems to be the wrong way round. Healthy activities and warm friendships are ignored. Destructive behaviour and damaging relationships are sought out. True friends – who wish nothing but the best – are treated as enemies. People who encourage further risky and unhealthy behaviour are seen as bosom pals.

In time the beneficial effects of taking things that 'work' in lifting the sense of inner emptiness are fewer – so they increase the dose or frequency – and the damaging effects become greater. Problems do not disappear. They mount up.

Eventually these addictive people find they can't live without mood-altering substances or processes but, because of the widespread damage, they also can't live *with* them. They are dependent on the very things that cause all the damage.

The previous excuses, justifications and rationalisations are no longer convincing to anyone other than people in similar fixes.

Families, friends, employers and well-meaning carers of one kind or another despair. Healthcare professionals become confused over why obviously sensible advice is ignored. They resort to inappropriate – or even insulting – diagnoses such as 'personality disorder'. Anything other than consider that an *addictive nature – a genetic predisposition* – may be at the back of all this mayhem.

And families go along with that. They see addiction as a disgrace, a weakness of will, a stupidity or even a depravity – something that happens in other families and in different parts of society. They blame *external* circumstances – anything other than accept that the problems go with the individual as well as with the environment.

Politicians and medical professionals also tend to be reluctant to see that some people have addictive natures. That diagnosis seems fatalistic.

But, without an accurate diagnosis, appropriate treatment cannot begin.

Alice (35) was brought to see me by her father. Addiction was not seen as a major problem. Various consultant specialists had provided a range of diagnoses: dyslexia, autism, Asperger's Syndrome, ADHD, Borderline Personality Disorder, You Name It. Her father said the real problem was lack of concentration, obstinacy with strong likes and dislikes, and fear of any change in plans. He described his daughter as being clumsy and untidy and having poor money management.

All that might apply to any lost soul. But then a more specific picture emerged: obsessive behaviour towards drinking, binge-eating and making very ill-advised relationships.

Chapter 2: Diagnosis

Accurate diagnosis – not over or under – is essential.

Terry Pratchett, who wrote the *Discworld* novels, described a character as being born two drinks short. He tries to catch up but gets the dose wrong.

Wow! Terry Pratchett got that absolutely *right*.

In Hazelden, the first rehab in the world, the psychologist Dr Richard Heilman uses the same definition of alcoholism in more scientific terms: the inability to predict what will happen to further alcohol consumption in any day after taking the first drink.

Ethyl alcohol is a mood-altering chemical. In some people at some times it acts on the mood centres of the brain, stimulating a craving for more.

This unpredictability is what Dr Heilman emphasises. 'We drink because the car turns left. Out of the blue, on a beautiful day, it turns left all on its own and stops outside a bar. And then we find ourselves drinking again.'

That's pretty well all the science we need to know in order to understand alcoholism, the brain illness that leads lovely talented people to become tyrants who destroy their families, friends, colleagues and everyone else around them.

We can study brain biochemistry and learn about dopamine reward pathways and other features of neurotransmission, in which one nerve cell communicates with another. But that doesn't help the counsellor or the patient. All it does is to get counsellors a certificate that satisfies employers. They are less likely to get sued for malpractice if they can show that their counsellors have been trained and assessed properly in 'best practice'.

That is defined by academics. They teach statistics and research methods but are unlikely to be able to show their students how to comfort, encourage and inspire. Those skills are not in their repertoire. They can't be assessed in examinations that lead to professional qualifications. So they tend to be ignored, dismissed or even feared.

But they're what patients need, what gets them well and keeps them well. They have to be attracted towards something rather than frightened away from something.

The most effective counsellors are people who are addicts themselves. They understand the problems from the inside.

I'm an addict. I believe I was born with an addictive nature. I haven't used addictive substances or done addictive things for over 30 years. But I'm still an addict. I could relapse back to my former behaviour if I become slack in maintaining my daily recovery programme.

Consider this: I'm short sighted. I was born that way. My parents were short sighted. My brother is shorted sighted. I wore glasses for 50 years. They enabled me to function. But at the end of that time I was still short-sighted. Wearing my specs day after day had not changed my eyes.

Having a chronic illness is not what we vote for. We like appendicitis rather than diabetes. We want an expert to take charge, go in, come out and finish. We don't want to be told that we need to take responsibility for ourselves.

Only 60% of patients with diabetes, high blood pressure or asthma carefully follow the recommendations given by doctors. Addicts are not the only people who want an easier, softer way. We're not the only stubborn mules on the planet.

But one particular problem that addicts like me have to learn about is the psychopathology of denial. A basic feature of addictive disease is that *it tells us we haven't got it.*

Nobody denies having a broken leg. It's obvious and we have a lot of pain. Being an addict is also obvious and it causes a lot of pain – mostly *to other people.* But tell any addict that he or she has an *addiction* problem and there will be a clear response: – "No I'm not – and anyway we're all addicted to something".

My own eating disorder could have been diagnosed when I was seven. I fell off a punt when I was sucking a lollipop. I went down into the water but I was still sucking the lollipop when I came up. It didn't matter to me if I drowned but I wasn't going to lose my lollipop. Sugar was what life was all about.

In adult years my weight used to vary by 50 pounds. I could take off excess weight by dieting and exercising but then I'd put it all back on again.

I shopped and spent for England, not for things I needed.

I took on work I didn't even want to do.

I smoked 30 cigarettes a day when I was the junior doctor on a heart ward, with patients all around me dying of cigarette smoking-related conditions.

I lost three months' income on the turn of one card in a poker game. And I went back the next day to try to win it back. I didn't. I lost more.

Through my compulsive helping – doing too much for other people and not enough to protect myself – I caused a lot of self-righteous damage, patronising and belittling other people when they could often do things perfectly well for themselves.

I had a whole raft of addictive behaviours. And many painful consequences. But my denial was total. I simply didn't see what was obvious to everyone else.

Even when my wife, Meg, was sitting in front of a divorce lawyer, I asked our family doctor what was wrong with *her*. After all, I paid the mortgage and provided for the children. What more did she want?

But I was in pain. I didn't want to lose her. That pain – the gift of desperation – is what turned me round.

I asked for help and was put into a side room in a private mental nursing home that housed 17 old ladies. My room was completely blank. There were no pictures. I had no telephone. The only window faced a brick wall five feet away. I had no visitors, not even the consultant psychiatrist who put me in there. The only person I met was the lady who brought my meals.

After three days of sensory deprivation I was going quietly mad.

But the truth was that I **was** mad – insane – already. I had been for a long time. I did my work as the senior partner of a major medical practice and I earned my living. But I was nuts. I had lost my sense of proportion on what mattered and what didn't. And I couldn't see that.

My head sometimes tells me lies. The devil is in the 'sometimes'. I don't know when.

Many years later, when I built my rehab, I employed counsellors who were like me – addicts who no longer took addictive substances or did addictive things. We know our patients' problems from the inside. We can't be hoodwinked by them. We've made the same excuses, told the same lies. And we know how to comfort, encourage and inspire them to get the spontaneous, creative and enthusiastic lives we have now.

Sidney (45) is an 'A' list celebrity. And he knows it. He has come to believe his own publicity material. After all, he wrote it. He was referred to me by a rehab director. Sidney had refused to get involved in group therapy. He is too important for that sort of nonsense. He knows what is wrong with him. He has 'stress'. It descends on him like a dollop of something. And it sticks.

He couldn't work or even leave his home. I saw him at his home just once, to establish contact. But, after that, in a great performance, he had to come to me. I do my work in my professional environment. That's where I function best.

He told me his life story. I sensed he had told it before to many people, many times.

Looking at his various issues in a new light was not something he wanted to do. He already knows all the answers. He doesn't need to ask questions. Or be challenged in any way. He's stressed and that's that.

In due course I joined his long list of people who don't understand his problem.

Chapter 3: Accuracy

When the 'more' button goes on, that's it.

My work focuses on helping people who *want* to be helped. That's fairly straightforward. But they may have fixed ideas on *how* they want to be helped.

They tend to want to learn how to drink alcohol sensibly rather than give it up.

They want to give up heroin and maybe acid and ecstasy but still use cannabis. They see cannabis as harmless, the social alcohol of a young generation.

Or they want to continue to use cocaine as a party drug they can take or leave.

Or they want to stay away from betting shops after the big win. And still continue to do the lottery. Increasingly.

Or they want to manage their weight problem with diets and exercise rather than accept they have a chronic eating disorder.

They do want to give up smoking. But not yet. It would be too extreme. They'll try vaping because they still get the nicotine hit. And, after all, they have to be addicted to *something*. Giving up everything would be too extreme.

So what I say is that they can try whatever they want and see if it works.

With alcohol I suggest they have two drinks at lunchtime every day for a week. They must drink that but nothing alcoholic before or afterwards. They reply that they'll give up altogether for a week. They know they can do that. They've done it before. And for longer. It proves to them they're not alcoholic.

But it doesn't prove anything to me. For an accurate test they need to stimulate the unpredictable 'more' button in their brains by having the two drinks at lunchtime and see what happens then. If they can remain abstinent without going up the wall in frustration, they probably do not have an addictive nature. But if they come back with a load of explanations – the celebration they had to join in, the business opportunity they had to lubricate, the friends they have to keep – they have a problem. The very problem they dread facing up to. They could be alcoholic.

This prospect annoys them because they see alcoholics as people who are in a far worse state than they are. Alcoholics don't have regular work. Alcoholics are abusive. Alcoholics sit on park benches, clutching a precious bottle of rotgut. A diagnosis of alcoholism is an insult.

Or druggies, hooked on one drug after another, reassure themselves that they can't be 'real' addicts because they're not on heroin. And if they are on it, they're not on much. Or they don't use needles. Not every day.

There is always a reason why the boundary between normal sensible use and addiction lies the far side of where they are. And when they do cross that boundary, they point to other 'not yets' in their behaviour.

Similarly, there are food addicts who see their problems as being rooted in the abuse and abandonment of their childhoods. Or in their metabolism. Or in the way foods are marketed. Or in anything other than in themselves, in the way they're made. And, by using health foods and vitamins, they keep themselves healthy. Don't they? And they've never done anything illegal. Not like real addicts.

Or the gamblers on property or stocks and shares who see themselves as investors, taking a balanced view on market movements. That was the intention anyway. Until the stupid government made a mess of things as usual.

Or the sex addicts who got lucky. Or found a way to live without really working. Or maybe they're working in a way they have a right to choose.

None of these people sees that he or she has a problem with addiction. The problem is in the outside world. Lots of problems. Not in the inside. Each of them makes his or her own choices in life. And they all feel free.

Except that they're not. They're obsessed with proving to themselves, and to other people, that they're not addicts.

But people who don't have addictive natures don't have to prove anything to anybody, least of all to themselves.

Addicts reassure themselves on whatever it is that they use as their particular mood-altering substance or process. Or when they use it. Or how. Or where. Or anything. But the thing they need to look at – if they have any hope of arresting their rake's progress and turning it round – is *why* they use it.

They tend to say they use mood-altering substances and processes because – obviously – they feel good when they do so. They tend not to see what happens after that. As a Chinese proverb says, 'First the man takes the drink. Then the drink takes the drink. Then the drink takes the man'. And that same principle applies to any addiction.

But if people don't believe they have a problem, they see no reason to ask for help. I myself do not have diabetes. Therefore I don't take insulin. And I'm not an addict so I don't need help in any way other than to have a bit of guidance on sensible use. The first statement – that I do not have diabetes – is true. The second – that I'm not an addict – is untrue. But it took me 47 years of painful experience to recognise that. And even then I wasn't really convinced. Even now, more than 30 years later, I still need reminding day by day. I'm insane. But at least I can be made aware of that now by recognising other people like me. And I can do something, day by day, to keep myself on an even keel and have the life of my dreams.

I had to recognise that my various addictions had specific characteristics in common:

1. Preoccupation with use or non-use.
2. Contentment with use on one's own.
3. Use primarily for mood-altering effect.
4. Use as a medicine, as a tranquilliser, antidepressant, sleeping tablet or pain-killer.
5. The need to protect the supply.
6. The inability to predict what will happen after the first use in any day.
7. Initially having a higher capacity than other people.
8. Continuing to use despite damage.

9. Continuing to use despite the repeated serious concern of other people.
10. 'Drug'-seeking behaviour.
11. 'Drug'-dependent behaviour.
12. The tendency to cross-addict, coming out of one addictive behaviour and picking up another.

Having any four of these addictive characteristics indicates the need for further assessment into the possibility of having an addictive nature.

That's bad news and good news. Bad news because it's the last thing we want to hear. Good news because, with clear differentiation between addicts and non-addicts, we can do something positive to end the self-delusional behaviour and put a stop to the torment.

Johnny (28) was one of the lads. "You ok?", he asked everyone else. It never occurred to him to ask himself the same question. Cocaine and alcohol were his real friends. He knew lots of people. He was in a 'people' business. He was happy. Determinedly so. But his wife and children were not. His occasional use of prostitutes was just a man thing. Until he ended his life permanently when the pain and shame were too much. And when the prospect of changing his values was overwhelming.

Chapter 4: Questionnaires

Addictive characteristics are precise, not made up by doctors or journalists.

The purpose of a questionnaire is to differentiate one population from another. Answers to an addiction questionnaire have to show who has an addictive nature and who does not.

It is as dangerous to give false reassurance as it is to over-diagnose addiction, saying that some people are addicts when they are not.

Doctors, sociologists and journalists love to make up their own questionnaires. They have their own ideas on what makes an addict and they stick to them.

They come up with questions such as, 'Have you ever had a drink in the morning?'. Night-shift workers drink in the morning. Priests serve Holy Communion in the morning. Ask a silly question and you get a silly answer.

Or they ask about variations in body weight. People with bulimia keep their weight constant. They can binge as much as they like but then they starve, exercise or purge. They may become habituated to using laxatives to ensure that food goes straight through them rather than gets converted into fat.

In questionnaires, drug addicts are unlikely to tell the truth on how they get and spend money. The Registrar General's *Abstract of Statistics* show how much the population spends on alcohol, tobacco, drugs and gambling. But these figures are sometimes overlooked by people who are concerned that government welfare payments are inadequate. A bizarre joke among drug addicts is

'**Question:** What's green and gets you high?
Answer: A Social Security giro cheque.'

My questionnaires have to be headed with, '*Have you ever?*'. In this way an addictive nature is revealed, rather than obscured by self-reassuring temporary abstinence.

The search for magic fixes is endless. As with addicts who say,

"We want what we want when we want it and we want it now", a chemical solution to a human spiritual problem has attractions for many researchers. But addiction is addiction, regardless of whether a particular mood-altering substance is legal, illegal, a prescription medication or a food.

Questionnaires are dangerous instruments. They have enormous risks when given too much credibility.

But they can be very valuable when pinning down specific populations – which, of course, is precisely what addicts don't want. And there are as many doctors, psychologists and journalists who are addicts as there are in any other sector of the general population. Addicts will tend to seek employment in places where they can hide their predilections. They become publicans or salespeople or anything where legitimate expenses can be massaged to accommodate their genetic drive for mood-alteration.

And researchers, doctors and journalists inevitably become interested in the subjects that most affect them in their personal and family lives.

I did that myself. My family is riddled with addiction in one generation after another. We're very good at it. But not all of us are affected. Maybe some did not inherit an addictive gene or lacked the traumatic experiences to cause it to be expressed.

So we need to look at large populations and determine which specific characteristics separate the addicts from the non-addicts. That was done in Chapter 2. Now we need to formulate questionnaires that are based solely on those addictive characteristics. For example, using primarily for mood-altering effect might generate the question, "Have you ever kissed a bottle of wine and told it you loved it?". Not all alcoholics would say "Yes" but no non-alcoholic would ever do so.

It should be clear that the twelve features of an addiction that I have listed are all – quite specifically – addictive characteristics. They are not exaggerations of normal civilians' behaviour. They are exclusively the behaviour of the addict foot soldiers in our continuing war with ourselves.

My questionnaires in total are self-validating. Any outlet in which there are no positive answers indicates no addictive tendency in that outlet. But it confirms the addictive nature of an outlet where there are positive answers – because the questionnaires are all based on the same twelve addictive characteristics. Clinically, I find that more than four positive answers in any outlet indicates the need for further assessment of addiction. That's the cut-off point.

Generally the questions should be answered for *lifetime use,* rather than making an assumption that previous use is no longer relevant. That addictive outlet may simply be resting and waiting to be reactivated. The extent of an individual's total addiction indicates whether he or she has any addiction at all or, perhaps, simply the need to be recommended to attend one or another Anonymous Fellowship and work the Twelve Step programme or, possibly, has a need for intensive treatment and extended care.

The answers to the full set of questionnaires on my website – real-recovery.co.uk – will show precisely where individuals have addictive tendencies and therefore where they need to be abstinent. It should be noted that depression underlies *all* addiction, and self-harming and obsessive compulsive disorder are aspects of *all* addictive behaviour. In some people these particular outlets are taken to extremes.

This corresponds with some people who have eating disorders becoming massively obese or dangerously thin.

My experience of looking after over 5,000 in-patients in my rehab over 23 years leads me to believe that addictive outlets come in three clusters. Each of these clusters may be determined by a single gene. For this reason it is important to be abstinent from all outlets in which there is one addiction. The gene needs to be switched off in order to prevent one addiction leading to another within the cluster and causing a relapse. This explains why nicotine addicts have twice the rate of non-smokers in relapsing back to using alcohol or drugs.

The clusters my researchers and I formulated are:

'Hedonistic': alcohol, recreational drugs, prescription drugs, nicotine, caffeine, compulsive stealing, sex and love addiction, computers, gambling and risk-taking.

'Nurturant of Self': food (bingeing, vomiting, starving, purging), self-harming, shopping, spending, work, and exercise.

'Relationships': relationship addiction (using other people as if they were drugs) and compulsive helping (using oneself as a drug for others).

Some people have outlets in just one cluster, some in two and some – like me – in all three.

My questionnaires, asking 10 questions on each of 23 addictive outlets, are based entirely on the twelve addictive characteristics. So much so that addicts often say to me, 'How did you get inside my mind?'. My answer is that I have the same mind: an addictive one.

Here are four of the questionnaires:

Alcohol
1. Do I find that feeling light-headed is often irrelevant in deciding when to stop drinking alcohol?
2. Do I find that having one drink tends not to satisfy me but makes me want more?
3. Have I had a complete blank of ten minutes or more in my memory when trying to recall what I was doing after drinking alcohol on the previous day or night?
4. Do I use alcohol as both a comfort and strength?
5. Do I tend to gulp down the first alcoholic drink fairly fast?
6. Do I have a good head for alcohol so that others appear to get drunk more readily than I do?
7. Do I find it strange to leave half a glass of alcoholic drink?
8. Do I get irritable and impatient if there is more than ten minutes conversation at a meal or social function before my host offers me an alcoholic drink?
9. Have I deliberately had an alcoholic drink before going out to a place where alcohol may not be available?
10. Do I often drink significantly more alcohol than I intend?

'Recreational' (street) drugs
1. Do I particularly enjoy getting a really strong effect from recreational drugs?
2. Do I have a sense of increased tension and excitement when I know that I have the opportunity to get some drugs?
3. Have others expressed repeated serious concern about some aspects of my drug use?

4. Do I find that getting high tends to result in my going on to take more drugs?
5. Do I tend to use drugs as both a comfort and strength?
6. Do I often find that I use all the drugs in my possession even though I intended to spread them out over several occasions?
7. Do I tend to make sure that I have drugs, or the money for drugs, before concentrating on other things?
8. Do I get irritable and impatient if my supply of drugs is delayed for ten minutes for no good reason?
9. Do I tend to use more drugs if I have got more?
10. Do I use drugs before going out if I feel there might not be the opportunity to use them later?

Food bingeing

1. Do I tend to think of food not so much as a satisfier of hunger but as a reward for the stress I endure?
2. Do I tend to use food as both a comfort and strength even when I am not hungry?
3. Do I find that being full is often irrelevant in deciding when to stop eating?
4. Do I find that I sometimes put on weight even when I am trying to diet?
5. Do others express repeated serious concern about my excessive eating?
6. Do I prefer to eat alone rather than in company?
7. When I have eaten too much do I tend to feel defiant as well as disappointed in myself?
8. Do I prefer to graze like a cow throughout the day rather than ever allow myself to get hungry?
9. Do I have three or more different sizes of clothes in my adult (non-pregnant if female) wardrobe?
10. Am I aware that once I have consumed certain foods I find it difficult to control further eating?

Compulsive Helping (Submissive)

1. Do I tend to pride myself on never being a burden to others?
2. Are others concerned that I am not doing enough for my own pleasure?
3. Do I try to avoid upsetting other people, almost regardless of the consequence to myself?
4. In serving other people, do I tend not to count the costs even though they mount progressively?
5. Do I tend to remain loyal and faithful regardless of what I may

endure in a close relationship?

6. Do I like to make myself useful to other people even when they do not appreciate what I do?
7. Do I tend to take on more work for someone close to me even if I have not finished the previous batch?
8. Do I feel like a real person only when I am performing services for someone else?
9. Do I often help someone close to me more than I intend?
10. Do I feel most in control of my feelings when I am performing services of one kind or another for someone else?

Julie (53) looked at the pie-chart print-out of the results of the questionnaires on my website and was very surprised. She knew she had a problem with alcohol – just a bit of one – but she wasn't prepared to see her cigarette smoking portrayed as an addiction rather than as an irritating habit. And she didn't like the idea of having an eating disorder, rather than a bit of trouble with her weight. And she was very upset with the idea of being labelled as a compulsive helper. I pointed out to her that I had merely asked the questions. The answers – labels if she liked – were hers. She didn't like that at all. She shot the messenger. I didn't see her again.

Chapter 5: Selling

How to sell an idea to people who don't want it.

Salespeople know how to get people to buy things they don't need and weren't aware they wanted. That's a macabre skill.

I try to sell addictive people something they clearly need – abstinence – but don't want. Not at any price. For this reason I am very often their last port of call, when they have tried and failed with other approaches.

Addicts have only one motive when they come to see me. They want to get out of pain. They change their behaviour only when the perceived pain of staying as they are is greater than the perceived pain of changing.

Ideally they want other people – family members or the government – to get them out of pain. And, by that, they mean getting someone else to pay for the consequences of their behaviour and take actions that will reduce future risks.

Alcoholics want their spouses to lie to their employers, saying they are ill.

Drug addicts want their family to find the best lawyer to get them off a charge.

Cigarette smokers want the state to take responsibility for the consequences of their behaviour when they themselves have not done so. They want taxpayers to pay for their medical problems.

People with eating disorders want understanding on the difficulties they have in deciding what to eat or not.

Gamblers want debts to be paid off before the heavies move in.

All these people tend to hate me when I suggest to their families that leaving addicts to get the consequences of their behaviour is the best course of action for the long term.

Without the pain there will be no gain. Future crises will be worse, and they will occur more frequently if addicts avoid experiencing the consequences of their own behaviour.

How many times does "Just this once" have to be heard? How many more promises will be made and promptly forgotten once the heat is off? How many lives will be damaged or even lost when good intentions are insufficient and while the concerns of family and friends are ignored despite all that is given?

I'm tough because I'm in a tough business. As a family doctor in South Kensington, I looked after a relatively young population. In 23 years in my medical practice I had 10 deaths. In that same time I had 230 deaths when patients did not follow the advice given to them when they were in my rehab.

That's a terrible toll. But it would have been even higher if the rehab had not existed. Addiction is a killer. Suicide is often the mode of death when addicts find they cannot live with or without their chosen mood-altering substances or processes on their own terms.

I see the primary function of a rehab as helping people who would be unlikely to get well any other way. And, as the head of the counselling team in the rehab, I saw my prime responsibility as reducing the relapse rate of patients. I'm always hungry for new ideas and methods of treatment. If people think something works, I want to know about it.

However, I'm not overjoyed at being told about ideas I first heard over 30 years ago and know, from very painful experience, don't work in practice.

For example, the idea that addiction stems primarily from abuse and abandonment in childhood, and that 'multi-generational shame leading to co-dependency' is at the root of it, is a very old idea. And it's very popular even today. I heard it, eloquently expressed at a sell-out conference last month. Anyone can sell that idea. It enables addicts to blame other people for their pitiful state, while sometimes giving lip-service to acceptance of the family's frailty.

To be clear on this, my name is Robert and I am an addict. My addictive behaviour goes with me. Irrespective of previous distressing experiences in my life, it's up to me to furrow my own path by following the example of those who have ploughed it successfully before.

Selling that idea is not easy. All I can do is talk about what my life used to be like in my days of active addiction, what specific changes I made, and what my life is like now. Then it's up to other people to decide if they want to do the hard work that I have done in turning my life around and keeping it moving forward one day at a time.

Some do. Some don't. But at least I've been honest with them by selling ideas that I can clearly demonstrate work in practice. I don't sell snake oil.

Thomas (56) is a lovely man but he has a rotten illness. When he works at all, he works hard and creatively. He's a gentle soul. To everyone but himself. When he gets drunk he is maudlin and self-pitying rather than abusive.

Selling him the idea that he – or at least his illness – is the architect of his own misfortunes has been a challenge. I listened at length to his story. We did trauma work, I showed him what I do to keep myself in reasonable physical, mental and emotional shape each day and I gave him a work-book that I find helpful. (I should do. I wrote it myself from my own experience.)

He was genuinely very grateful. And he went on drinking.

His wife is in despair. How can an intelligent, sensitive man be so self-destructive? so arrogant? so incapable of following simple suggestions?

The answer is that this is the nature of the beast. I can sell *him* my ideas but his addiction doesn't buy them.

A civil war is waged inside him between the man and his illness. When he fights himself he loses and he gets hurt.

I'm seeing him and his wife next week. I wonder when he will feel that he's had enough pain for one lifetime. Maybe now. Who knows?

Chapter 6: Causes

Genes, environment, and exposure.

As I see it, there are three causes for addiction.

The antecedent cause is genetic. Some of us are born that way. We can say dammit and we can fight against it but that changes nothing. We are what we are.

Then the contributory cause is trauma of one kind or another. This wakes up a craving for mood-alteration. Somehow.

Finally, the precipitant cause is exposure. We discover something that works for us in lifting our mood and we use it.

All three of these causes have to be present for addiction to take off.

My wife, Meg, had a dreadful childhood. But she inherited her mother's compulsive helping rather than her father's primary addictive nature. Meg had no primary addiction at all. She drank alcohol occasionally for the taste. She didn't smoke, use drugs or have an eating disorder and she didn't gamble.

I had an odd childhood but not a particularly abusive one. I had the sexual abuse and bullying that was customary in British private schools in those days. Maybe it still is. Anyway, I don't believe I suffered any more than any other boy. And boarding-school separation from parents was a common experience just after World War II. Parents were still in the forces or in the diplomatic service or in business or they were missionaries, as mine were. I was well looked after by my guardians. They survived me, rather than the other way round. I was dreadful.

Meg was lovely. Everybody said so. Many people couldn't understand why she married me. Yes, I shared her love of music. But my addictive behaviour was scarcely less abusive than my father-in-law's. In some ways Meg's compulsive helping and my primary addiction were a perfect fit. Her 'need to be needed' met my 'need to be fixed' in a 'co-dependent' relationship.

(By the way, this is the only sense in which I use that term. It tends to mean so many things – being equally addicted to several things, coming from an addictive family, being in a relationship with an addict, being abused or abandoned: you name it, someone will call it co-dependency – that it really means nothing at all.)

The childhood trauma that Meg endured was intense and repeated day after day from the age of four onwards. But it didn't make her into an addict of any kind. She lacked the genetic potential.

In my case, I clearly had the genetic drive. I ticked all the behavioural boxes even then.

An addictive nature can be diagnosed in childhood long before there is any use of mood-altering substances or processes. There are 12 characteristic features that apply:

1. Coming from an addictive family.
2. Feeling separate from other people.
3. Having wild mood swings for no obvious external reason.
4. Trying to control everything with reasons and excuses.
5. Being easily upset.
6. Being easily bored and frustrated.
7. Having a poor attention span (commonly diagnosed nowadays as Attention Deficit Hyperactivity Disorder, whereas I see it merely as a precursor of overt addiction).
8. Feeling lonely, angry, sad, misunderstood, picked on and resentful.
9. Not doing as well at school as previously.
10. Stopping activities that were previously enjoyed.
11. Getting into repeated trouble.
12. Picking new friends who also get into trouble.

(All these characteristics are illustrated on YouTube in my animated cartoon entitled *Preventing Addiction for Beginners*.)

I had all those characteristics, but the beginnings of my eating disorder were the only obvious signs of my underlying addictive nature.

As time went on I discovered a whole range of addictive outlets. I used them one after another or several at the same time. I always liked to keep a mood-altering substance or process in reserve in case my first choice was unavailable. Even though I had a very privileged adult life as a doctor, I had to have something readily available to change the way I felt at any time if I sensed the need to do so.

Meg had the same access to mood-altering substances and processes as I had. But she had no inclination to use them. I did. I was an addict right across the board, including in my own compulsive helping.

At the age of 70, Meg suddenly died of a stroke caused by a berry aneurysm, a weak-walled bubble on the side of an artery in her brain. She'd had it all her life. She'd had raised blood pressure for some years but who knows why the aneurysm burst when it did? The aneurysm was simply part of the way that she was made. So was her compulsive helping and so was my addictive nature.

Exposure to particular mood-altering substances and processes determines our specific addictive outlets. We didn't have alcohol to any great extent in any of my childhood homes. My parents and guardians couldn't afford it. And there were no drugs.

In adult life I carried morphia in my medical case every day of my professional life. But I never used it once. When I had an injection of Omnopon (a drug similar to morphia) for a gallbladder operation, I thought it was bliss, out of this world, sheer heaven. Clearly I have the potential to be an opiate addict or another form of drug addict. But fortunately I never went down that route.

All three addictive causes came together in my case but not in Meg's, other than in her genetic potential for compulsive helping.

I talk and write about my addictive nature with no sense of shame whatever. I'm not ashamed of my propensity to make gallstones and kidney stones. That's just the way I am. And the same is true for having an addictive nature.

I have lots of guilt over stupid, inconsiderate and hurtful things I've done in my life. I'm totally responsible for my behaviour in so far as it affects other people. I cannot hide behind my addictive nature and say, "I did that because I'm an addict". That would not be true.

I did not choose to be an addict but I do choose my behaviour and always have done. I'm responsible for it. I have to learn how to stop doing it. And I have to make amends to those I have harmed. Only then can I move on, be the person I want to be and live a life free from the clutches of my addictive nature.

It's still there but it doesn't control me any more. Through specific daily actions I keep my addictive potential in remission. I don't want to go round that loop any more.

I love the life I have now. My wife Pat and I have been married for five years and she has never known – apart from rare occasions in which I lose my cool – how awful I can be.

Freda (35) is a ball of anger. She bounces all over the place. Her cocaine addiction doesn't help. To nobody's surprise, she's going through her second divorce. I gave her a copy of my *Spiritual Awakening* workbook (I have no religious belief but I have a strong sense of the potential beauty of the human spirit seen in love, hope, honour, kindness, acceptance, forgiveness and other behavioural attributes.) She put it in the bin. That's her choice. Retrospectively, I think I should have waited until she asked me for it. I don't have the right to impose my values on her.

Chapter 7: Progression

Addiction progresses in a wavy path downwards.

We decay as we get older. I ran the London marathon when I was 50. I couldn't do that now. My spine is in enough trouble already from my osteoporosis (inherited from my mother, along with my eating disorder). I don't want to make it any worse by pounding the pavements.

My blood pressure is the same as it was in my twenties. My lungs and liver and kidneys, and other bits and pieces of me, are fine as far as I know. But I'm gradually going off. I know that. Inevitably. I'm not immortal.

My father's mind went to heaven three years before the rest of him. He died at 96. He had a good innings. Through his missionary work and time as a professor of mission and as a parish priest, he brightened the lives of many people, particularly when he wrote the Christmas pantomime each year. My mother was an artist, an illustrator of manuscripts, especially those of young men like her only uncle – a poet – who was killed in World War I. My parents were good people. All my family were.

I remember my mother's brother, my first guardian, saying that he wanted to make the world a better place for other people to live in. That wasn't compulsive helping. It was pure human kindness and he put it into practice as a socialist politician. I was privileged to be shown good values throughout my childhood.

But I betrayed them as my addiction got progressively worse as I got older. As with any other addict by the end of my using days, the only emotions I had left were blame and self-pity.

Each of my addictions had got worse. My eating disorder was out of control. I had given up smoking only because it caused me to get tightness in my chest. My gambling had switched from card games to property ventures. That meant that the risks – and therefore the addictive buzzes – were greater. My workaholism came out all over the place. I often took on work that I didn't want to do. But it wasn't until after Meg had died that I realised my own compulsive helping is probably the strongest of all my addictive outlets. Mine was overshadowed by Meg's. Perhaps I hid it or simply didn't recognise its full intensity while she was still alive.

But, one way or another, I was in deep spiritual trouble at the end of my using days. I was a mess.

If addiction progressed in a straight line downwards over the years, it would be easy to see it. Two or three points on a graph would predict the place of the next in the gradual disintegration of our mood, our behaviour and its damaging consequences.

But that's not the way it goes in addiction. The graph follows a wavy path. There are times when we are definitely getting better. Or, at least, not getting significantly worse. We use those times as reassurance that we don't have a major problem. People close to us often come to the same conclusion – encouraged by us to do so.

But then we fall off our secure perch and off we go again in our desperate search for a final solution. Anything to keep our spirits – and our bodies – alive. Somehow.

And so we resort again to our tried and trusted friends. Not human beings but the mood-altering substances and processes that worked before.

But this time they have less powerful effects. So we increase the dose. And the crises in our lives become more intense than before and they come more frequently. That's what shows on the graph.

The last thing we want in that situation is to be told by some bright spark that he or she knows what would be good for us. So on we go...

Julian (65) was a very distinguished physician, the senior consultant specialist in a teaching hospital. To protect patients from his alcoholism, his colleagues took away his admitting privileges. At that point, his family asked for my help.

Then, before I had seen him, they changed their minds, saying, "He's not all that bad". He was dead within a month.

Chapter 8: Hope

There has to be hope and inspiration.

"You know how it is, Charlie Brown", said Lucy. "You win some; you lose some". Charlie Brown, who had never won anything in his life, said "Oh that would be wonderful!".

I suppose I sell hope. I've got plenty. More than enough to share with others.

When my wife, Meg, died after we'd been together for 51 years, I didn't know what to do. I didn't want to live but I didn't want to die. I was bankrupt as a result of my incompetence in running a business and through a major fraud by my accountant. I had no idea how I could ever earn a living again or develop a productive life in any way. I was living in an old people's home in Canterbury, 70 miles away from my lifetime haunts in South Kensington. And I was separated from all my friends and my major interests. Canterbury is very nice but it's not my spiritual home. I knew I had to get back to central London somehow. Or die.

I handed back my corody, the document signed by the Archbishop of Canterbury that said I could stay in my tiny flat for life and the Church would pay my rent if I could not afford to do so. I had to make the jump *before* I had any idea where I would land.

But I had made similar jumps previously. I had resigned my medical partnership in the NHS group practice I created. I knew it wasn't going anywhere in terms of the development of ideas. The NHS is a top/down directed system. The government decides. The minions follow. That doesn't suit me. I'm always hungry for new ideas and new ways of doing things. So I jumped.

Four years later I resigned from the NHS altogether, losing my guaranteed income and the part-payments for the costs of my staff and premises and also my further NHS pension rights. When junior doctors on strike say they would go private if all they wanted was more money, they have no idea what they're talking about. Fee-paying patients expect service. They don't open their wallets and say, "Help yourself".

When I established my rehab, by mortgaging everything we had, I lost £1,000 a day on it for a whole year. That's a lot of money now. It was a fortune in 1986.

But I survived each of these jumps. And subsequently survived bankruptcy and bereavement. My resource is in my experience and in my ideas, not in the bank.

I know that if my life is going nowhere I have to jump first and then, in the new situation, work out where I might go next. To take the easy option of staying put – I was very secure and well paid in the NHS when I was 33 – would have killed me. I would have betrayed my creativity.

I have hope based on very real experience. I know how to survive. I know how to have peace of mind in spite of unsolved problems. I know how to make happy and mutually fulfilling relationships. And I know how to be spontaneous, creative and enthusiastic. These are my daily goals. They're written out on a whiteboard in my rented office.

I did that in order to show my counselling patients today that material goals can be destroyed in a moment by political turmoil. But spiritual goals cannot.

By the time patients come to see me they are in the same spiritual mess I was in when I got to the end of my using days.

That's why I tell them my personal story. I have no need to tell it for my own therapeutic reasons. Not 33 years after becoming abstinent, eight years after losing my professional base and seven years after losing Meg.

But I do need to show that I know how to come through exceedingly difficult times and move on.

When people are in the trough of despair and cannot see beyond the abyss, they need hope.

They cannot get that from pious platitudes, heartfelt homilies or intellectual instructions. They need to know, from someone who has done it, that *it is possible to come through.*

I recommend new patients to watch YouTube clips of Byron Katie. She tells her story of being incarcerated in mental hospitals, stuffed full with medications, or stuck in bed at home, for ten years, unable to move forward spiritually or even physically. Yet now she gives international audiences a sense of hope that they can move on by doing what she calls 'The work'.

This involves asking themselves three questions about their most negative belief:

1. Is it true?
2. Is it *really* true?
3. *Who* (not what) would I be if it were not true?

She inspires millions through giving them a sense of hope.

I also suggest to my patients that they watch YouTube clips of Alice Sommer Herz, a Holocaust survivor. At the age of 108 she was playing the piano and giving lucid interviews.

These two amazing people – and others such as Father Joseph Martin, whose *Chalk Talk* on recovery from alcoholism is on YouTube, Governor Harold Hughes who introduced The Hughes Amendment to The Constitution of the USA that confirms alcoholism as an illness, and Geraldine O Delaney (wonderful initials!) who was still running a rehab in her 90s despite the relapse and death of her husband – inspire me. They, and many others – such as Hal Marley, the USA Drug Tsar who always spoke of developing "an attitude of gratitude" – inspire me to this day. Memories of my brief times with all these people give me hope for the future, whatever it brings. I'm merely handing on their message.

Also, right at the start of my time with my patients, I get them to write down a list of 10 things they're good at. This lifts the gloom and reminds them that – however low they've been brought by their illness – they still have talents that can be put to good use when the time is right. This gives them hope.

Amy (16) left school with no qualifications whatever. She told me there was nothing at all she was good at. I asked her what part of her life she enjoyed. "Hockey", she said. I asked her to write down 10 things involved in playing hockey.

She wrote
1. You have to be fit before you go on the pitch.
2. It's a team game.
3. You have to listen for commands.
4. It's strategic

and so on…

I looked at her list and commented that all she needed for a happy future was a skills transplant, taking talents she already had and applying them to other areas of her life. With her hockey skills – careful preparation, cooperating with others, listening to them, making careful plans and the rest – she could be Prime Minister if she wanted to be. Now she has hope.

Chapter 9: Action

The magic words are 'Do it the way that works'.

We don't get anywhere by merely thinking about goals. We have to define them and then do the necessary work to enable ourselves to achieve them.

I ask new patients how they would get from South Kensington to Kodaikanal. When they say they don't know where that is, I tell them it's where I was born.

I had asked them a question they couldn't answer. And then given them information they couldn't use. That, in my experience of much of it, is called 'counselling'.

It is only when I tell them that Kodaikanal is in South India that they can work out for themselves that they should go first to Heathrow, then to Mumbai, on to Madras and so on.

I use this analogy to illustrate that if we don't know where we want to get to in life, we won't know how to get there. We'll go here, there, everywhere, all over the place and never find what we're looking for.

But first we need to take stock of our values. An exercise I did for myself, and now recommend to others, is to write out a list of the 12 things I value most and another list of the 12 things I value least. Here are my lists:

I value most
1. The lives of my wife and children. They represent my primary choices and responsibilities.
2. My own life. I owe it to no one.
3. My principles by which I live my daily life. I do not borrow them from other people. I choose them. I would betray them under duress to save the lives of my wife and children, and my own life, but only if no innocent person's life would be lost in the process. I value my life and therefore I value yours.
4. My mind. I do things to enhance it and I don't do things that would damage it.
5. My health. I do things to enhance it and I don't do things that would damage it.

31

6. My creativity. My creative output confirms that I am alive.
7. My time. I choose what I do with my life each day.
8. My interests. I have the right to my own enthusiasms.
9. My profession. I have a professional responsibility to those who pay for my services in any sphere of my activity.
10. My friends (including some members of my family). My friends share my values. I develop new friendships as I myself change.
11. My possessions. I am entitled to the product of my labours.
12. My country. I would fight to protect our common culture of tolerance.

I value least
13. My reputation. I judge myself by my own values.
14. My knowledge. I have more to learn.
15. My achievements. Some of them were fine – but they are past.
16. My seniority. Respect should depend upon behaviour, not upon age or length of tenure of a position.
17. My status. I have none. Therefore I have nothing to lose. My talents, such as they are, go wherever I go. I alone am responsible for the flowering of my natural ability. No other person, and no social position, can give me a sense of personal value.
18. My physical prowess. This would be a ludicrous value.
19. My 'cool'. Individuality has substance. Fashion has none.
20. My professional group. Those I respect are counterbalanced by those I do not, as in any other profession. I set no store by my particular profession. Take away my daily enjoyment in my work and I would find another profession.
21. My political group. I have ideas of my own and do not accept that might is right. Mere numbers may produce no more than the lowest common denominator. There are, in any case, more constructive occupations than scoring points off opponents.
22. My financial group. My values are determined by what I believe, not by what I can purchase.
23. My family as such. I have no obligation of family ties to those with whom I share few values.
24. Life after death. I'm too busy and happy in this one.

With continuing experience, I can change these values at any time. They're *my* values, no one else's. I wrote them out in 2002. I haven't modified them at all since then. But I could.

My suggestion is that each one of us should write out our own lists, not that other people should follow mine.

My values determine my daily actions. I do what I believe in. I don't do things I don't believe in. For example, I shall never again work for the state. I don't believe in collectivism in any form. I fear it. My experience has been that it destroys individuality and creativity, the most precious aspects of our lives.

On the other hand, I value money as an honest means of recognition of value in exchange of goods and services, but I have no interest in accumulating wealth for its own sake. I bought property for the purpose of providing services to patients.

I know what I want in life. I want to be free from the stranglehold of my addiction. Without that freedom I am an automaton, driven towards self-destruction and damage to others.

I want to contribute something to other people, and to the world in general, through my counselling work, my writing and broadcasting and other creative activities.

I want to do anything I can to heal wounds and join people together rather than cause pain and separation.

I judge myself on my actions. If something doesn't produce the result I look for, it is not a useful behaviour. I make no judgement on whether the behaviour was good or bad, right or wrong. If it doesn't get me what I want it isn't *useful*. I therefore change my action and the idea upon which it is based.

In moving on from my days of active addiction, I've had to change many of my values and actions. They drove me into blind alleys of arrogance and self-centredness. I don't want to be that person any more.

I believe I was born with an addictive nature. But I don't do addictive things nowadays. Through the plasticity of my brain tissues, I am able to shape myself into being the person I want to be. All I have to do is to take simple positive actions day by day by day by day by day.

Ben (25) – because of his age – knows everything about everything. I was the same in my teens and twenties. He doesn't see that he might benefit from re-evaluating some of his concepts and attitudes. He knows that cannabis isn't addictive, that old people should make way for the young, that there will be a new millennium when we have the right government. He knows it all.

I tried – gently – to show him that I know something he doesn't know. I know how to get clean and stay clean, free from all addiction and free to choose whatever I want to do in order to be happy, creative and productive. But it's up to him to decide if he wants to share these values – some of them maybe – or carry on as he is and get the inevitable consequences.

Chapter 10: Consequences

Addiction always gets worse. Pain is the teacher.

If a man has lost his job, lost his wife and lost his driving licence, it is probably superfluous to ask about his alcohol consumption. There are few other ways of acquiring those consequences.

Addiction has consequences in every aspect of life: behavioural, medical, social, financial, professional, marital, everything. No other illness does that. Cancer doesn't. Diabetes doesn't. Heart disease doesn't. Even ALS, which Stephen Hawking suffers from, doesn't.

And, in a separate category, poverty doesn't. There are many poor people who live very dignified and positive lives. As a family doctor in North Kensington, I saw that every day.

Widespread consequences can therefore be used as an approximate diagnostic test for addiction.

Social instability is also a rough guide. Addicts tend to drop through the social strata. Their priority is their addiction. That's where they spend their time and money. When they can't afford any longer to live where they are, they move to somewhere cheaper or set up a squat. The end result of that movement is that deprived areas have a disproportionately high number of drug users. But the problem goes primarily with the individual, not with the environment.

These addicts develop a sense of entitlement. Benefit cheques belong to them by right. They do not have to thank the taxpayers who provided the money. Nor even the government who administered it.

Give a man a fish and he eats for a day. Teach him how to fish and he eats for life. Give his community a load of subsidised fish and you destroy the business of the local fishmonger and you give people a sense that they deserve to be fed for ever by someone else. That is an addictive attitude and practice, a barbaric one, not a compassionate one at all.

Strangely, Robin Hood is usually portrayed as a hero. He was a lazy good-for-nothing thief and rabble rouser. He should have earned his living and then chosen what to give away from his own resources.

Praising him – and thieves who become political tyrants – indicates a very weird philosophy and morality, an addictive one, believing in control and domination while disregarding the individual rights of other people. Nowadays the 'human rights' lobby tends to fight for the rights of everybody other than hard-working and contributing members of the community. But that's politics.

Addiction and politics overlap on the issue of legalisation of drug use. The most damaging of all addictive substances are nicotine, sugar and alcohol. In the UK nicotine kills 300 people a day, sugar 200 and alcohol 100. (Multiply by 5 for the USA figures.) Yet these substances are all legal. Put together all the illegal drugs – heroin, cocaine, acid, ecstasy, speed, cannabis and the rest – and they kill 50 a day.

At first sight this looks as if young people are right in saying that cannabis is merely the alcohol of their generation and that the legal drugs are far more dangerous than the illegal ones.

But it could be that use of the illegal drugs would become far more widespread if they were to be legalised. The experience of Colorado and Washington State following legalisation of cannabis would appear to bear out that fear. Consumption has rocketed and so have the damaging medical consequences.

The idea that legalisation of drugs would get rid of the bad guys is fanciful in the extreme. There is nothing the Mafia would like more than to be seen as legitimate businessmen.

My own suggestion, until now, is that drugs should be de-criminalised but not legalised. People caught using illegal substances should be sent by the courts to rehab rather than to prison. This means that addicted users will get the treatment they need and occasional users will get a wake-up call.

The same principle should be applied in schools. Users, and even dealers, of illegal drugs should be sent to rehab and then taken back into the school afterwards. Of course there would be a parental outcry that dreadful addicts – let alone wicked dealers – should be let back into a school and be a risk to other children. But that view is short-sighted.

The children in the school already know who the drug users and dealers are. A policy of expulsion will cause this vital resource – the awareness of other children – to clam up. A policy of re-introduction after rehab would result in children wanting to help their friends.

But will schools take on that policy? Not in my experience. When I suggested it 20 years ago in the Deputy Heads' annual conference, each school was reluctant to be known as a druggie school. Ha! They're *all* druggie schools. The question is which of them want to do something positive about that and help the children rather than worry about their own reputation.

And on the issue of responsibility, how responsible is it for schools to have a lax – almost encouraging – attitude towards consumption of alcohol on school premises by senior pupils?

Alcohol is a social lubricant but it is also a major killer and destroyer of families and businesses. I am no prohibitionist. But I do advocate finding out who has an addictive nature – my questionnaires do that from a very early age – and intervening appropriately when help is clearly needed.

But will schools and parents accept that it is reasonable to ask questions about family problems with alcohol and drugs and eating disorders alongside the questions that are asked about cancer, diabetes, asthma and heart disease? I doubt it.

And that means we're stuck as we are, with inconsistent laws that are openly resisted and flaunted. And the whole of our society gets the consequences of that.

Mary (38) woke up one morning and found a strange man in her bed. In shock, she turned away – and found another. She remembered nothing of the previous evening from the time she left to go to a party. She thought it might be sensible to ask for my help.

Chapter 11: Self-Esteem

We feel good when we do good things in line with our values.

Family members often tell me that the addicts in their lives suffer from poor self-esteem. My experience is the opposite. Addicts tend to be grandiose. They live in permanent adolescence, believing themselves to be the centre of the universe.

At the same time they wallow in self-pity. Sigmund Freud described this dual state as 'king-baby', His Majesty must be obeyed but the baby needs to be nurtured.

In addicts the sense of self is utterly self-centred. They learn any number of subterfuges in their determined quest to avoid uncomfortable feelings. Their goal is to close down all bad feelings but keep the good ones. That cannot be done. We are either sensitive or we are not. But at the same time, by suppressing feelings, addicts become emotionally fragile and touchy.

No wonder the Facebook world is littered with emoticons. When words are inadequate, from lack of skill in using them and lack of clarity in identifying a feeling, an emoticon or a ghastly 'sticker' – a thumbs-up sign or a waving hand or a shower of hearts or frowns – is imposed upon the reader's attention.

Young children, trained by peer-group pressure to communicate in this way, see little need to learn any other.

The behaviour of addicts can be described accurately as 'adolescence writ large'. Most children grow up, take the world as it is and interact with it appropriately. Addicts do not. Like adolescents, they are determined to change the world rather than change themselves.

Everyone builds castles in the air but addicts live in them. They don't want to face reality. They want to bend it to their will. Then they spatter their distorted feelings in all directions in order to prove to the world how sensitive they are.

But they confuse two meanings of 'sensitivity' – being sensitive to other people's feelings and being conscious only of their own, being prickly, easily hurt and frequently offended.

Addictive substances and processes provide good feelings on the cheap. They give an instant artificial high or blandness or whatever other feeling is preferred. Bad feelings can be avoided. Good feelings don't have to be earned. That artificial emotional world suits adolescents and addicts very well. Addicts are often described as being "25 (or 35 or whatever age they actually are) going on 13".

In adult life most of us learn to use our feelings as indicators of the appropriateness of our behaviour. When we do bad things we feel bad. And when we do good things we feel good. Addictive disease – even before the use of mood-altering substances and processes – distorts this natural process. Addicts want 'good' feelings all the time and they don't want 'bad' feelings at any time. They reject the need to *earn* their self-esteem and the respect of others; they *demand* it.

I want to feel *all* my feelings. I want to feel sad so that I can also feel happy. I want to feel lonely so that I can also feel the warmth of companionship. I need the contrasts in order to differentiate one feeling from another. And I want my self-esteem to be based on something tangible.

Most people try – unsuccessfully – to base their self-esteem on achievements, comparisons and associations.

Passing an examination or winning in sport is only that and nothing more.

And so what if one is better than someone else at something? Is that the best one can say for oneself?

Meeting a 'celebrity' is fine. But did that person remember you?

Any achievement, comparison or association can be bettered at some time by someone else.

The use of stimulant drugs and steroids and all sorts of other chemical aids in sport is cheating. It is widespread because applause and adulation are felt as primary needs by those fraudsters. They don't want genuine competition. They want the prize without having to earn it.

That's exactly what addicts want.

To rely on achievements, comparisons and associations for one's self-esteem is odious. Celebrity worship is pathetic. Who cares about the political views of a singer? or the personal opinions of sports people or television 'personalities'? The answer is that a great many people do. The tabloid press and tv gameshows feed that monster.

I value *all* human beings equally. As a family doctor I saw them come into the world equally fragile and, for the most part, leave it equally frightened – but I do not give their viewpoints equal validity. I listen when a genuine point, rather than a mindless rant, is being made. I know that progress tends to come from the periphery rather than from the centre. Ten years experience – on a committee or some-such – may mean nothing more than one year's experience repeated ten times. I learn from mavericks and odd-balls, addicts even. I don't respect the views of place-men and women.

I'm not naturally conservative in my views. I am unashamedly – proudly – elitist in wanting to deepen my understanding. Active addicts are not. They already know all the answers. Why should they ever ask questions?

Addicts specialise in talking drivel. 'Turn on, tune in, drop out' was the counterculture-era catch phrase popularized by Timothy Leary in the swinging sixties. And a fat lot of good that idea did him or his hippy followers. They finished up indistinguishable from each other, clones rather than individuals. That's no achievement at all.

Comparisons have to take privilege of birth and opportunity into account. After that there may be little to crow about.

Associations are an attempt to gain vicarious self-esteem. I once met Princess Margaret. I shook her by the hand. As a small boy alongside my father, I was in a queue of people waiting to greet her when she named a new ship for The London Missionary Society. Does my meeting her give me some knock-on significance? Ha! I fear not. But if Princess Margaret had gone back to the palace to tell her sister that she had met me, that might have been something. But somehow I doubt she did.

And that brings us right back to the start in considering the self-esteem of using addicts. They have none because they have no individuality. They rely on other people for their sense of self. But when you've seen one active addict you've seen them all.

Self-esteem is an inside job. We create it for ourselves, based on our values.

Jilly (31) slept around a great deal when she was at university. It gave her a sense of being needed and wanted. Her eating disorder didn't help her self-esteem. She was forever trying to change her shape in order to influence the opinion she had of herself and, hopefully, the opinion other people had of her. It didn't work. She never developed the skills involved in learning how to make genuine relationships. She's a very lonely lady now.

Chapter 12: Chronic Illness

Once an addict always an addict – but we don't have to do addictive things.

Addiction is a chronic illness. Families reject that. Addicts resent it. Doctors, psychologists, nurses and social workers are disappointed by it. And politicians ignore it. They all strive to change the world so that addicts and other trouble-makers will learn to live in harmony inside their troubled minds and in the wider community.

Four ideas about addiction tend to be universal:

1. I'm not an addict.
2. Some people in my family, and some other people I know, have difficulties that need to be understood so they can be helped.
3. Addicts have had a bad up-bringing and have got in with a bad crowd.
4. I know absolutely what should be done.

By contrast, after many years of painful personal and professional experience, I have learned simply to say

1. I am an addict.
2. Various members of my family and some of my friends are addicts. I understand them very well but most of them don't want to hear what I have to say on this subject.
3. They were and are much loved and they were very well brought up, as far as I can tell, relative to other families I know.
4. I know I cannot help them. I'm too close to them.

Generally there is a belief that what addicts most need is love, education and punishment.

I've known thousands of addicts and I still work with addicts of one kind or another every day. I'm a long way from those know-it-alls who say 'I know someone who...' Addicts have often been very much loved in their childhoods. Because of their difficulties, they tend to have had a lot more time and attention – and they are often given more opportunities and more money – than their siblings. But that didn't change their addictive behaviour.

Love is fine. But it doesn't help an addictive tendency any more than it would help appendicitis.

Addicts have often been very well educated. I've treated addicts from some of the finest schools in the country as well as some of the worst.

I've given talks in many schools. I always introduce myself by saying that I may not look like an addict but I am. And even though I do not use addictive substances and processes nowadays, I still have an addictive nature. The pupils tend to ask for me to speak again. The teachers and parents are often not so keen. I didn't say what they wanted me to say.

I don't tell schoolchildren about particular illegal drugs. They know more about them than I do. I tell them I know I can't influence them but I know how to get clean and stay clean. They may know more about drugs than I do but I know a lot more than they do about addiction and recovery. That makes them curious and concerned – for their friends if not necessarily for themselves.

University students are more challenging. They know that the purpose of university is to use lots of alcohol and drugs, sleep around, and do just sufficient work to come out with a degree. They don't want me messing up their way of doing things. And after all, my own years at university were not exactly pristine behaviourally.

Trying to teach doctors, psychologists and other healthcare professionals about addiction and recovery is impossible. Doctors tend to like intellectual approaches – like Cognitive Behavioural Therapy – and they believe in prescribing pharmaceutical drugs. They're taught pharmacology. They trust it. They don't want to know about touchy-feely stuff. (For that matter, nor do I.)

I remember speaking to a group of 30 family doctors in a post-graduate centre 20 years ago. After my first sentence, saying we can't love, educate or punish addicts out of their addictive behaviour, a lady in the front row said, "I don't agree". She got up and walked out. I doubt that her experience of treating addicts – other than with substitute drugs and very sensible advice – was a fraction of mine. But she didn't want to know any of my ideas and that was that.

Punishment doesn't work in helping addicts to change their

damaging behaviour. They become cynically immune to it. I never changed my behaviour despite being the most punished boy in the history of my school. I held the records for beatings, detentions and copies, in which I had to write out 'Egypt for the Egyptians' three times to a line and 20 lines to a page. But no punishment changed my views or my behaviour.

I don't imagine that all addicts are like me. I don't believe that there is such a thing as an addictive personality. We each have our own personality even though we may share an addictive *nature.*

I have a public confidence but an inner personal insecurity. I'm at ease on live television – except for the necessary tension required to keep myself focussed – but I'm not keen on parties. I don't know what to say. In that sense I'm rather shy.

Other addicts are bubbly or brash. That's them, not me.

But we all share a sense of inner emptiness that has to be filled somehow.

The way we fill it is idiosyncratic. I use whatever mood-altering substance or process works for me. Recreational drugs have never attracted me. They frighten me. Gambling should have frightened me – my pulse certainly rose – but it didn't really scare me at all. I went on gambling for years after first getting into trouble with it. I simply got into bigger trouble.

But even that didn't stop me. I wanted the buzz. Like the fisherman who talks about the one that got away, I boasted about what I lost.

There is insanity of one kind or another in all addictive behaviour. Acknowledging that is the first step in redirecting our rake's progress.

Paradoxically, the three things that work in helping addicts to turn around are love, education and punishment.

The *love that works* is the love of one addict reaching out to help another to get well. The one who does the loving is the one who benefits. That is best done anonymously. When I'm doing my professional work, it doesn't count towards my recovery. In that situation I have a professional relationship with the addict. When I encourage and support a stranger – an addict, not anybody – I feel good. The inner emptiness is filled and I have no craving. Doing kind things for non-addicts does not have the same effect. It's a nice thing to do but it's not sufficiently specific to help me counter the urges – compulsions – of my addictive nature.

The *education that works* is the necessary understanding of addictive disease. As for many clinical conditions, some people have it and others don't. Those of us who are addicts by nature need to know about it. People who have friends or family members or work colleagues who have addiction problems – and that's a lot of people altogether in the general population – may benefit from this education but there's no need to cram it into everybody. Correspondingly, they don't need to know everything there is to know about cancer or heart disease or diabetes unless those conditions have some specific relevance for them.

The *punishment that works* is the punishment we addicts give ourselves when we finally recognise how dreadful our behaviour – and our lives in general – have become. I never, never, never want to risk going back to being the addictive idiot I used to be. I've had enough pain. And I've caused more than enough pain. I've tried to make appropriate amends for the damage I've caused. I don't want to cause any more. The rebound effects of my addictive behaviour on my peace of mind and self-image are too painful.

My illness is *chronic* and therefore my treatment, as for any addict, has to be continued indefinitely on a day-to-day basis. This is perhaps the most unpopular concept of all. People – family members in particular but also many healthcare professionals as well as addicts themselves – prefer to believe that detoxification is the only intervention required. Once we're clean we're clean. But that's true only in so far as it goes. And it goes only as far as the next disappointing relapse.

Confusingly, our personal behaviour (and often our physical appearance) may be at its *worst* when we are abstinent and craving for relief of withdrawal symptoms. When we give in to the craving and relapse, we are calm and content. In that state we may be greeted warmly with "Well at least I understand you now" – when the true situation is not understood at all.

Long-term recovery has to be founded upon long-term acceptance of the need for long-term treatment. The helpful short-cut is for us to imagine that we're doing it only for today. Then, as Scarlet O'Hara said at the end of 1,024 pages of *Gone with the Wind,* "Tomorrow is another day".

Alf (40) is a recurrent patient. He lives in a revolving door. He's been in treatment, in one rehab or another, again and again. He came to see me six months ago after I hadn't seen or heard of him for years. He asked me whether he should have another bout of treatment. I said no. He already knows all that I would be able to teach him. And he's been theraped to hell and back. He doesn't need any more. His recurrent problems come from failing to put into practice each day the things he's been taught for years.

Chapter 13: Problems

Of course we have problems. Everybody does. But we learn to live with them.

There's a wise saying that we should be careful what we wish or pray for. We might get it.

I was careful when I wrote a book of prayers for atheists and agnostics. Just as The Salvation Army don't see why the devil should have all the best tunes, I don't accept that believers in religions should be the only people to have wish lists.

My prayers are psychological reminders to myself that I can have the life I want if I think carefully about it and if I take the actions most likely to bring these wishes to fulfilment.

Here's the prayer I wrote for June 20th:

I can't get the government off my back.
I can't borrow money from the bank except when I don't need it.
I can't do what I want without adequate resources.
I can't rely upon all professionals to deliver a professional service.
I can't persuade children to write thank-you letters and turn down their music.
I can't teach the dog to behave politely to visitors.
I can't remember when life did not have one problem after another.
Dear God, help me to remember that a life without problems would be indescribably boring.

Active addicts want a life free from problems. They don't tolerate challenge or emotional uneasiness at all well. They want instant gratification of their wishes. Waiting is purgatory.

The problem is they don't learn from experience. They keep doing the same things they did before but hope they will get different results this time.

In my counselling work, I know that in order to help people to get well, I have to make them *insecure* in their beliefs. Otherwise they will continue the same behaviour as before.

Addicts tend to believe that something must be good for them – or even vitally necessary – if it makes them feel good. This is a fundamental misconception. Things that make them feel good artificially are bad for them because they fail to learn the true effects of an experience.

I remember a young man saying, "I feel better when I take Ritalin (a stimulant drug prescribed for Attention Deficit Hyperactivity Disorder). That means my body needs it". That is the same as alcoholics saying alcohol must be beneficial because they feel better when they drink. But, sadly and frighteningly, doctors often make the same mistake as this young man. They believe that their treatment methods must be effective if patients say they feel better on them. That is a disaster. Many patients are prescribed treatments that make them worse rather that better, despite the initial response.

So-called 'antidepressants' are very damaging. As mood-altering drugs, they are addictive to people who have an addictive nature. The effects are gradual and cumulative. It takes two weeks for the initial positive effect to be felt. And it also takes two weeks for withdrawal symptoms to be felt if the drugs are suddenly discontinued. But, by that time, the doctors say that the recurrence of symptoms clearly indicates that the drugs were necessary in the first place. So they put the patients back on the drugs that were the cause of the withdrawal symptoms. That is an exact parallel to alcoholics using 'the hair of the dog' – another drink – to settle their 'hangover' symptoms of withdrawal.

The tragedy is that these difficulties are all avoidable. There are better ways of dealing with problems than by ignoring them, suppressing the symptoms they cause, or using pharmaceutical or recreational drugs (what's the difference as far as the brain tissues are concerned?) to escape from reality.

I don't want a life in which my feelings – such as they would be – are in hock to the pharmaceutical industry. I am familiar with love and hate, hope and despair, tranquility and turmoil. I want *all* of that. Not some bland 'blah' in which mere interest has displaced passion.

In my residential rehab all our patients were depressed. That's why they were there. After the initial five to ten days of detox, if at all necessary, we used no drugs other than Vitamin B6 (Thiamine), multivitamins and medicines to prevent withdrawal seizures. We knew from our own experience that there has to be a substitute for the mood-altering substances and processes but this does not have to be chemical. It can be *behavioural*. After all, there are many mood-altering behaviours – shopping, spending, work, exercise, sexual activity, gambling and risk-taking and many others – so there is nothing essential in chemical prescription. The body makes its own antidepressants.

I believe addiction should be termed 'neuro-transmission disease'. That gives a precise label to the genetic defect that leads to addictive behaviour.

There are genetic defects in every organ of the body. It should be no surprise that the brain, the most complex organ of all, should also have genetic defects.

In the thinking part of the brain we are familiar with many genetic problems. Perhaps Down's Syndrome is the best known. It would be extraordinary if the feeling part of the brain – the mood centres and their interconnections – did not also have genetic defects.

I believe the innate sense of inner emptiness that all addicts – of any kind – feel is due to a chemical defect in the way one mood cell in the brain communicates with another. Scientists have already discovered many neuro-transmitters, the chemical messengers that are secreted by one brain cell – neuron – and picked up by another. The best known are Serotonin, Dopamine, Nor-adrenaline and GABA. I don't think it helps clinicians and counsellors to know more than that. We can leave it to the research scientists to let us know what they find.

The crucial issue is that the neuro-transmission system should be *expected* to go wrong sometimes in some people.

Imagine that one neuron sends six units of mood to another. If the synapse – the junction with another neuron – is faulty in some way, maybe only five units of mood arrive on the far side. So patients who have this defect feel a sense of being 'minus 1'. Understandably they are delighted when they discover substances and behaviours that have a 'plus 1' effect. So they use them. The most important point is that they're not looking to get 'high' but simply to feel *'normal'*.

I don't know what 'normal' is. I'm not a normie. I'm an addict. But I know when my feelings are bouncing around all over the place and I know when they are calm or stimulated appropriately.

Last week my wife, Pat, and I were at a magnificent performance of Wagner's opera *Tristan and Isolde*. We know this opera well. But we had never experienced such wonderful singing, acting and playing as in this performance in Longborough Opera.

At the end of the last football season, Tottenham finished above Arsenal in the Premiership League. That's good, very good. Pity about the knock-out Cup competition but things don't always go the way we hope.

What I'm describing here is the emotional effects of two recent experiences. No artificial chemical was involved. My own neuro-transmitters gave me a treat, two treats.

But my baseline is in a healthy place at the moment. I've done a fair amount of reaching out to help other addicts anonymously recently so my neuro-transmission systems are functioning well, despite me having all sorts of potentially worrying things on my mind.

The current political situation – nationally and internationally – worries me. So it should. But it doesn't lead to me hitting the bottle or the fridge or the casino or anything else. Nor did my bankruptcy and bereavement, nine and eight years ago. Reaching for addictive substances and processes at those times would have made things worse for me, not better. I know that from previous experience. I don't need to re-learn lessons I already know.

As a using addict, like others, I used to believe that the world had problems and I had solutions. Now I know that's the wrong way round.

Sylvia (26) had a difficult childhood and a difficult early adult life. Very difficult. Her father had been abusive and demanding. Her mother preoccupied and self-pitying. Her sister obsessed with one man after another. Sylvia escaped into drugs. But she discovered that she hadn't escaped at all. She took herself – and all her problems – with her wherever she went and whatever she did. So she got married. But her husband was also an addict. Their addictive behaviour was just about all they had in common. The marriage didn't last but the child did. As a single parent, drugged to her eyeballs, Sylvia decided that her son needed a better life than she was giving him. Her parents suggested she should have him adopted. Her sister didn't care what she did. Eventually, when I did EMDR (a psychological process that helps to put traumatic episodes into history) with her, she told me about 105 distinct disturbing events in her life. With great courage in the course of a month, she went through them all, one by one, until they no longer troubled her but were simply a part of her past. Now she looks after her son and gives him the stable environment he needs and deserves. And she herself is happy and at peace with the world for the first time in her life, even though I think she's a bit thin. Maybe she'll ask for help with that some other time.

Chapter 14: Futility

Much of the life of active addicts is futile. Recovery is creative and fun.

I ran my rehab at the same time as continuing to work as a family doctor. I had no choice. I had to earn my living from my medical practice. The rehab lost money – and always did – so it survived only when I repeatedly remortgaged it when property prices went up.

My medical colleagues were puzzled by me. I remember one asking me, "Why do you waste your time on those addicts? Just tell them to stop". Another said, "You're doing good work but it's not medical". I asked him if he would look for ways of helping people to stop smoking only after they got cancer of the lung. He didn't like being put on the spot like that by me. Our relationship didn't survive. While I saw his work as significant – he is an excellent doctor – he saw mine as trivial, misguided, futile.

With my particular feel for eating disorders – because I have one myself – I have looked after many patients who have had similar challenges. As the first person in the UK to put eating disorder patients into a rehab alongside people with alcohol or drug problems, I was mocked by my own treatment director. "Nobody's been caught thin or fat in charge of a motor vehicle", he said. Subsequently I was also mocked by the senior staff of a major treatment organisation – until they discovered that I had more patients in my care than they did. Then they offered my junior staff heaps of money to go to work for them. Some did. There was a time when all the counselling staff of one well-known rehab had been trained by me. I enjoyed knowing that. It meant that my ideas had taken root without me needing to buy the place. That's what I call a result.

I find it curious that doctors tend to be dismissive of rehabs – other than those where they simply give patients a comfortable bed, fill them up with drugs and then give them occasional 'group work' along with art therapy and classes in flower arranging.

As I see it, I was helping my patients to reduce their risk of getting 'real' illnesses, such as cancer, diabetes and heart disease, by getting them off the substances that would lead to them getting those conditions.

But other doctors tended to see me as a maverick. I have learned to wear that badge with pride. The only reputation that interests me is that I shall be thought to be a serious-minded professional.

Many of my contemporaries are retired or dying off. I'm not. I think the reason is that I've found an incredibly rewarding field of work. Most doctors start with patients who are in reasonable shape and then watch them gradually decay. I start with wrecks and work alongside them as they get better and better until they don't need me at all. At that end-point any further work I did with them would be unnecessary, futile.

Jonathan (65) has had a very successful life professionally. He still works as a money man in the City of London. And he's still married. When I first met him last year, all of that was at risk. It still is, of course, just as my recovery is. We can never afford to be complacent in our continuing recovery from addiction. But Jonathan's in great shape right now. I can see that. I hope I am too. But I'm not the one to judge. I simply do the necessary footwork each day to maintain my recovery as best as I can. Everything else in my life – including my marriage, my work and all my interests – depend on that. I can see Jonathan and he can see me. Perhaps it wouldn't be too futile if, next time we meet, I were to ask him how *I am*.

Chapter 15: Manipulation

Addicts are supremely crafty but have to learn to be open and honest.

An alcoholic will steal your money and sympathise with you in your loss.

A drug addict will steal your money and help you look for it.

A gambler will steal your money and ask you for more.

A foodie will steal 'in dire necessity'.

All addicts of any kind know how to look you straight in the eye and tell whatever lie suits their current purpose. They are well practised.

In the clash between behaviour and values, one compromise leads to the next.

Initially, when behavioural standards slip, there is a struggle to force them back into line with long-held values. In time it becomes less troublesome to adjust values to match the new behaviour. The boundary between acceptable and unacceptable behaviour is progressively shifted. Something that would never be done becomes an occasional event. Later it occurs daily. Justifications and rationalisations flow easily as the barriers of ethical standards gradually disintegrate.

The addictive behaviour becomes paramount. It is the primary driving force, above loyalty to friends and family. It disregards previous educational and social background and develops a counter-culture, seeking out others who share these new principles and attitudes.

Climbing back out of that spiritual cesspit is an immense challenge. Civil war rages inside the head of each addict in the tightening grip of addiction. The residual quiet voice of the human being says, "Help me". And the insistent harsh voice of the illness says, "Get away from me". Inevitably the louder voice takes precedence.

Only in time, as painful consequences mount up, is the quieter voice heard at all. Even then the harsh voice is insistent that it must be heard above all others. In this way we come to understand that our addiction wants us dead. It is a parasite that has no care at all for the host on which it feeds.

The brain has selective memory. To move something from short-term memory into long-term memory requires structure and repetition. Years down the line we can remember poetry we learned at school. But we cannot repeat word for word the talk we heard yesterday. As a medical student I had to learn to split my mind so that I could listen and take notes at the same time. As an addict I learned how to say one thing but do another without betraying any sense of contradiction.

In the use of mood-altering substances and processes, I would remember the initial good feelings but forget the subsequent crash. As with other addicts, I would try subsequently to re-capture the good feelings. I wanted an immediate hit. Despite all previous experience, I didn't even consider what would happen after that.

Bailing addicts out of the painful consequences of their behaviour is therefore counter-productive and dangerous. They *can't* – not won't – hear personal concern and sensible advice. They learn to reconsider their determined addictive behaviour only when they imagine that going on as they are will be more painful than changing.

Of course there are risks in letting addicts take the consequences of their behaviour. But the risks of not doing so are greater.

Judith (54) and **Jeremy (58)** did not despair of finding a way of persuading their elder son, **Paul (30)** to change his behaviour. They had no need to do so. He had done well at school. He had probably drunk a bit more than was good for him but nobody – certainly not the teachers or the school doctor – seemed to be at all concerned about that. At university he got introduced to cocaine. He fell in love with it. He found the sweetheart he had always dreamed of. He didn't see that he could possibly be addicted to it because it was just a party drug, not something he took every day. In any case, his work didn't suffer, so nobody – least of all his proud parents – were concerned about him. In due course his cocaine use became more frequent and – at the end of a smart dinner party – someone passed round some heroin to combine with the regular cocaine to make a 'speedball'. It felt good and it didn't seem to cause any immediate problem. So Paul convinced himself that all the scare stories about drugs – and heroin in particular – were overrated and he was sensible enough, tough enough and mature enough to look after himself. None of that turned out to be true. But it was his younger brother, **Tom (27)**, who expressed concern. When Paul didn't listen, Tom was in a dilemma. Should he tell their parents about his concerns? He decided this information – given to him by a mutual friend – was too important to keep to himself. Judith and Jeremy were horrified and decided it couldn't possibly be true. They were glad to be reassured by Paul, who then turned on Tom and said their relationship was over. For ever.

Chapter 16: Control

The pipe-dream of addicts is to be in control. Healing comes through recognition of powerlessness.

Addicts talk of being, 'wasted', 'out of it', 'smashed', indicating these as pleasurable states. They like knowing that they are interfering with the complex, delicate functions of their brain tissues. Even when told that these symptoms indicate that they are damaging their most precious body organ, they continue their behaviour as before (after making crude remarks).

Smokers sometimes refer to cigarettes as 'cancer sticks' – as if macabre humour makes their behaviour acceptable. In effect they are saying to themselves, "It's my life. I'll do what I want with it". More accurately they might say, "My addiction is in control of my life". I haven't smoked in over 40 years. I don't want to continue to damage the delicate alveoli (air sacs) of my lungs or fur up my arteries. But, more than that, I want to experience my own feelings, rather than suppress them.

And, as far as all other mood-altering substances and processes are concerned, I have no wish whatever to be 'wasted', 'out of it', 'smashed' or anything else in that self-destructive lexicon.

I like my mind as it is. It does what I ask it to do. It thinks clearly. It reasons and ponders. It can be awe-struck or amazed – without any artificial stimulus.

I love the sight of my wife's smile, the smell of new-mown grass in the Square, the taste and texture of blueberries, the sound of a top rate jazz band, the warmth of the overcoat made from cloth my uncle gave me, the awareness I have of vibration, position and balance. I love everything I experience through the interpretations my brain gives to sensory signals.

And I love the movements that I can make. My osteoporotic spine hasn't crumbled away altogether. Not just yet. I'm in pretty good shape generally because I keep myself fit with daily exercise. My body still obeys most of the signals my brain sends it.

I like all the things my brain does for me.

And I like to feel in control of my mind and therefore also of my body. This doesn't make me a control freak. Quite the reverse. It gives me freedom to choose.

Throughout today my mind has been active and in good nick. I have no wish whatever to be greeted by an acquaintance with, 'Robbertt, Yourenofunnowadaysh'.

Patrick (45) came to Meg's memorial service. It was kind of him to think of her and me. I would have preferred him to be sober but that peaceful inner state was not in his gift. I know that.

Chapter 17: Fear

The unknown is fearful but it can be exciting when we can see the benefits.

Addicts of any kind ought to be frightened of what they are doing to their bodies and minds by using mood-altering substances and processes. They're not. They're worried by the prospect of running out of their supply or of having to give up altogether.

They're used to suppressing their feelings. A rehab joke is that the good thing about recovery is that we get our feelings back; and the bad thing about recovery is that we get our feelings back.

Families, on the other hand, tend to do a lot of worrying on behalf of the addicts. I remember a father telling me that he was fully aware that his son knew the combination number to the home safe. The father deliberately put money into the safe so that the young man could steal it and get his money for drugs that way rather than by stealing it from someone else. I explained to the father that he was maintaining his son's addiction rather than helping him to get off it.

That was not persuasive. The father's greatest fear was that his son might be caught and get a criminal record or be sent to prison. He did not take kindly to my observation that this might be a good thing if it was the painful stimulus that might lead towards getting him into recovery. Being unable to get a visa to enter the USA, or being incarcerated in prison, are better outcomes than finishing up in the morgue.

Understandably, the greatest fear of family members is that the addict might get into serious trouble with the bad guys or might die. But they tend to go the wrong – ineffective – way about trying to allay those fears.

The mother of a potential patient of mine paid off his gambling debt of £100,000 when he told her about the threats he had received. She didn't think it was necessary to do anything further. He had promised her he wouldn't gamble again. The pressure was off and there would therefore be no further stress and no need for treatment of any kind. Hmm…

Families often want me to identify tablets and other substances that, fearfully, they find in their children's rooms. Most of all they want to be shown samples of various addictive substances and paraphernalia so they know what to look for.

I think that's a disastrous course of action. Suspicion, fear and control become the basis of family relationships from then on. It's not a good way to help children to be honest about their behaviour and get them to ask for help if they are in trouble with addictive substances and processes. It poisons relationships rather than nurtures them.

I understand the parents' fear only too well. I've had it myself and many of my worst fears came true. It was an exceedingly difficult time for Meg and me. Today our elder son runs a rehab. That's the best possible result of our intervention into his addictive behaviour.

Despite being a doctor, I had very little knowledge about addictive drugs. I had not been taught about them in university – nor about addiction as such, rather than merely about its medical consequences – and I had never used them. But I was able to observe my son's general behaviour, note its progressive decline in standards and observe its consequences in every aspect of his life. That's a far more reliable method of finding out if someone's taking illegal drugs than invading privacy by scrabbling around looking for them.

Discovering whether children or adults are using other addictive substances or processes follows the same principle: observe the changes in behaviour and note the damaging consequences in all aspects of life.

And count the spoons.

Bella (31) has an eating disorder. At school she had become obsessed by her body weight and shape. Putting on two pounds, and not being able to get into size 10 – let alone size 0 – clothes would be a catastrophe. That's not particularly worrying. 60% of girls in their teens have similar concerns. And they learn from each other how to burn off calories through exercise, repeatedly clenching and unclenching their buttocks, throughout the day and half the night, unobserved by anyone else. And they learn how to enforce vomiting by sticking a couple of fingers, or a toothbrush, down their throats.

But that doesn't mean they have bulimia nervosa as such. They are just girls in that age group.

A man told a genie that his one wish would be for world peace. The genie thought that would be too challenging. He asked if the man had any other wish. "Understanding my teenage daughter" was the reply. The genie stroked his chin and then said, "Let's talk about world peace".

Bella couldn't be criticised. She was top of her class in almost all subjects. As far as her parents were concerned, she was the best girl in the world. When she subsequently turned to compulsively overeating after giving up the unequal battle with the tape-measure and scale, they noticed the increase in weight. Her mother – as a friend – commented on it. And on her over-spending. World War III broke out.

Chapter 18: Intervention

How do we stop the ones we care for damaging themselves and other people?

In the 1960s Dr Vernon Johnson, in the Johnson Institute, spelt out a technique for intervening in addicts' behaviour. No longer would addicts have to 'hit rock bottom' and lose everything before turning their lives around. 'Rock bottom' had been below the mortality line for many of them. They died rather than give up their mood-altering substances and processes.

If that isn't proof of addicts' determination and willpower, I don't know what is. Addicts are frequently thought to be inadequate and weak-willed. Nancy Reagan advised "Just say no". Betty Ford, the alcoholic wife of another president, knew better. She founded the world-renowned Betty Ford Center that treats alcoholics and drug addicts through the Twelve Step programme first formulated by Dr Bob and Bill W, the co-founders of Alcoholics Anonymous.

When I visited the Betty Ford Center I was told that they don't treat eating disorders and other addictions – other than cigarette smoking – because they don't want "to confuse the message". I observed that they had patients with eating disorders in front of them but they weren't treating them.

Even today I get told by some self-defensive alcoholics and drug addicts that I'm not a 'real' addict because I didn't hit 'rock bottom' in *their* particular way. My rock bottom was more spiritual than physical. I was washed up emotionally. I'd come to the end of my tether in my relationship with myself. I looked into the abyss of suicide and didn't like what I saw.

Nobody else intervened in my behaviour in a formal sense. Meg said that she didn't want to live with me any more. And then, by chance, I had a fortunate insight.

A patient of mine in my medical practice asked me if a particular drug she had been prescribed was 'mood-altering'. I had no idea what she meant. She explained that she was a recovering heroin addict and that drugs that altered her feelings might cause her to relapse. I said she couldn't possibly be a heroin addict. Her father and I were at Cambridge together. And anyway, what did 'recovering' mean? If she was no longer taking it, she'd cracked it. She corrected me, explaining that she was abstinent because she worked the Twelve Step programme of Narcotics Anonymous. I asked if that meant she held hands under Waterloo Bridge. On hearing that I'd never been to a meeting of NA or AA or any other Anonymous 'Fellowship' as these groups are uncomfortably termed, she suggested I might go to one before making any more wisecracks.

So I went to one in the Red Cross centre in Old Church Street, Chelsea. And I met three patients of mine. I asked them why they hadn't told me about their addiction problems. Surely, as their family doctor, I needed to have that information. What followed was one of the most formative statements of my professional life:

"We couldn't tell you, Robert. You're a doctor."

I resolved to become the sort of doctor addicted patients *could* talk to. After all, addicts of one kind or another cause immense damage to themselves, to other people and to society at large. If I could help them to get clean and stay clean, I would be doing something far more significant, clinically and socially, than writing out prescriptions and certificates and giving 'sensible' advice.

So I began my journey into my own recovery and into learning about setting up and running a rehab. Since then I've travelled all over the world, visiting rehabs, attending conferences and giving talks.

I remember speaking at a Non-Governmental Organisation conference in Hong Kong. I put across the ideas of addictive disease and recovery. The speaker after me, a consultant psychiatrist from London, said that he was discarding his prepared speech in order to spend his time saying how wrong my ideas are.

In Kent, where I built my rehab after spending weekends there for 20 years, the medical director of the local alcohol services said "If you had told us your plans we would have told you not to come here. You and your ideas are not wanted in this area." The head psychiatrist in the local hospital said "Private practice is against God's law". A fellow of a college in the University of Kent at Canterbury (where I am an honorary fellow at another college) attacked me in an article in *The Times* and spoke against my ideas in a public conference in London. As the first questioner after his talk, I asked how he could be so critical without ever meeting me or visiting my rehab which was only 20 minutes away from Canterbury. I invited him to come to see us at work. He never did.

Despite all that hostility from professional colleagues, I was warmly welcomed by the local population. After Pfizer Pharmaceuticals, I became the largest employer in East Kent, even bigger than Hoverspeed, the hovercraft company in Dover. But when I spoke to Locate in Kent, a government-sponsored body charged with increasing employment in the area, I was told that this does not include private medical services. I explained that I had left the NHS because I would not be allowed to innovate, put new ideas into practice. I had had no choice but to mortgage my home and office and set up a private organisation. He was unmoved.

These various critics didn't want to know. Maybe I should have used a modified form of the Johnson Institute intervention techniques on them. (Incidentally, I see from the web that the Johnson intervention is now depicted as the *cause,* rather than preventer, of deaths from addicts hitting 'rock bottom'.)

These techniques – evolved from the significant personal and clinical experience of the specialists in the Johnson Institute – are to say to the addict

1. I love you (or I'm concerned about you)
2. AND (*not* 'but' – because that would cancel out the love).
3. I observe... list 3 facts that cannot be denied. Give no opinions.
4. I recommend... Give a clear statement that gives no alternative choice. Otherwise addicts will duck and dive, choosing their own advisors and therapeutic approaches.
5. If you do not agree, I shall... (Never make a threat that you are not fully prepared to carry out.)

When I said all this to my son, he said, "That's a helluva choice, Dad". I replied, "Yes: yours".

I once had the privilege of meeting the Nobel prize-winning economist, Professor Friedrich Hayek. "My boy", he said (I was 50 at the time), "never try to influence your contemporaries. Wait for them to die off!"

I understand his humorous advice very well. I have to accept rejection of my ideas as a fact of life. But I'm still trying to influence other people through various media outlets, both mainstream and social, and through writing this book and others. And I remember only too clearly how dismissive I was of Twelve Step ideas when my medical practice patient first told me about them.

Anonymous (age: too old), a senior member of the British Medical Association Inner London Local Medical Committee of family doctors, said to me, "When you've been a member of this committee for as long as we have, we might consider looking at your ideas". I resigned.

Chapter 19: Knowledge

Adults know a great deal about the wrong things.

As I've said before and will again, you can't teach people who already know. I myself enjoy *not* knowing. I like finding out new ways of looking at things. Factual knowledge is interesting but new concepts and practical considerations fascinate me. I want to learn where I am wrong so I can get better ideas and see how they work out in practice. Sycophants who agree with everything I say are no use to me. I learn nothing from them. My friends – including my wife, Pat – challenge me.

I believe that if the solutions of today could solve the problems of today they would have done so. We have to look for new ideas and ways of doing things if we are to move forward.

The idea that addiction is an illness is not new. Resistance to that idea is not new either. This resistance comes primarily from a very narrow concept of the words 'illness' or 'disease'.

People accept that heart disease is an illness. They also accept that it has a mixture of genetic and lifestyle causes. They think the same about cancer, diabetes and asthma. They also understand thyroid deficiency and other hormonal conditions, deficiency states and the effects of age and decay. They understand infections. And, of course, they understand trauma.

When it comes to mental illness of any kind, the situation is more confused and often contentious. The concept of an illness of the human spirit would be unlikely to enter any determinedly secure head.

Doctors resent 'their' words (illness or disease) being appropriated by non-medical people. And they often tell me – forcibly – that addiction is *not* an illness:

1. It's self-inflicted. (Would they refuse to treat sports injuries?)
2. It's a personal responsibility. (How about contraception?)
3. It's a social problem. (How about unemployment?)
4. It's an emotional problem. (How about bereavement?)
5. It's self-limiting, burning itself out in time. (How about virus infections?)

6. It's untreatable. (How about Huntingdon's Chorea?)

Doctors may try to justify their ownership of the words 'illness' and 'disease' in these ways – and refuse to treat addicts of any kind for these reasons – but, as I hope I have shown, their concepts – and therapeutic ideas – do not go deep enough.

In most clinical fields the understanding of doctors is clear and reasonable. But not always. A criminal psychopath does not see that torturing or murdering someone is wrong. The issue of criminal responsibility is therefore one for psychiatrists and lawyers. So far so good.

The age of adult responsibility varies from one issue to another. People in England can marry and serve in the armed forces, but not vote, at 16. That's a bit confusing. Patients in mental institutions are not considered by Social Services to be adult until they are 18. That's definitely more problematical.

In my rehab I was required to provide specific services for 'children' who were very much 'adult' in some of their behaviour. Drug addicts know the ways of the world long before the age of 18. At the extreme, I remember a 14 year old – the youngest age I was allowed to treat – telling me she wanted to get off drugs and give up prostitution, to which she had been introduced by her mother when she was 11. Evidently they used to do double acts together.

Psychiatrists, psychologists and social workers knew what 'should' be done for her but very few tried to do it. My juvenile addiction unit was one of only two in the country. They've both gone down.

In my residential rehab I remember being challenged on not providing sufficient supervision for detoxification of a particular patient. As ours was not a secure unit – we had no fences keeping patients in and visitors out – I could not stop her collecting drugs when she wanted them. Addicts can always find whatever they want and they can always find ways of paying. Nor could I give any explanatory information to the family member who expressed the concern. The patient was over 16 and therefore an adult entitled in law to confidentiality.

In London the authorities who had responsibility for supervising my extended care facility, where patients came for follow-on care after their initial treatment in the rehab, decided that our patients needed to be treated on the same principles as residents of old people's homes when new regulations on room sizes came into force. (There were no written standards for 'halfway houses' like ours.) My wife Meg and I lived in the basement while 12 patients – and 24 feet – lived above us. Our children had left home by then so there was plenty of room in our former family home. But the authorities decided that our patients needed to have 12 square metres of floor space for single bedrooms, 18 for double rooms and 24 for triple rooms. I pointed out that our patients were generally young and fit. For much of the day they were out on educational courses, in part-time work or using the local swimming pool and tennis courts. The total number of square metres in our halfway house was the same as would be required in an old people's home. I had simply divided the space between bedrooms and living rooms in a way that was appropriate for our patients. This argument was not accepted and – after five clinically very successful years with excellent outcome figures – we had to close. We had lost money even on full occupation. We certainly could not afford to lose one third of our beds, as we would have to do to meet these requirements. The end result was a bureaucrat's dream: the regulations were kept intact but there were no patients to supervise. Ours had been the only halfway house in the borough. The juvenile unit closed as well, for slightly different bureaucratic reasons.

I am not against regulations in care homes. There have been far too many abuses. I am simply saying that common sense needs to be applied rather than total inflexibility. But try telling that to people whose own jobs – and pension rights – depend upon ticking all the right boxes!

So I'll say it again, as promised: you can't teach people who already know.

Steve (40ish at that time) had silver eyes. I knew him in the old days when I was an active member of the North Kensington Labour Party. He looked straight through me when he talked about 'The Cause'. He knew absolutely what he believed in. I was more impressionable. He frightened me. Later on in my political journey, when I wrote the speech for David Penhaligon, the Liberal Party Health Spokesman, to give in the 'pay beds' debate in the house of Commons, the leader of the party, Jeremy Thorpe, said to his colleagues, "Right. That's the speech. Now, which way shall we vote?". They didn't appear to me to have clear ideas at all. Further on again in my undistinguished political career, I became a Libertarian. I left that group when I saw no liberty in the use of drugs, as some of the others demanded. And that was the end of the story for me. Nowadays I play no active part in politics at all. But Steve? God knows.

Chapter 20: Experience

Learning how to stop and stay stopped comfortably is the art of recovery.

Throughout this book I have given examples of my personal and professional experience. This is the background from which I write.

It is very clear to me when writers or speakers lack this vital experience. What they write or say does not ring true. It reminds me of an orchestral musician damning a particular conductor by saying, "He knows a lot about music but he's not a musician".

Laboratory knowledge of the physiological effects of mood-altering substances or processes gives no insight whatever into *why* someone would take them. Statistics are about numbers, not individual people. They are of value to epidemiologists studying the breadth and spread of a clinical condition. And they should be useful to politicians making plans for the distribution of resources. But they are of no value to a clinician like me, working face-to-face with an individual patient.

Professor Geoffrey Stephenson, the Emeritus Professor of Social and Applied Psychology at the University of Kent at Canterbury, was chosen by me to be the head of my research department. I needed him and his assistant, Nicholas Zygouris, to let me know if my ideas were working in practice for our patients over time. I also listened to their suggestions on what approaches might work better than those I was already using.

It was Geoffrey who introduced me to the work that has been done on motivation and stages of change. He also suggested that Mindfulness meditation techniques might be useful for our patients. But I wouldn't ask him to run a group. As a normie, and even as a psychologist, he would not be able to spot the subterfuges and games that addicts play.

I know them because I've played them. In my using days I was able to change sides – in the middle of a discussion – without Meg even noticing. I remember my treatment director describing a particular patient as being so slippery he could slide under a door without taking off his top hat. I was thinking of both of them yesterday when

Pat and I went to see the musical *42nd Street*, which my treatment director and I had seen in New York. Twenty-five years down the line, I'm still regularly in touch with both of them. They had style. They still do.

And early yesterday morning, at a meeting, I sat next to another patient from those days and was greeted by yet another who was over from France for the week. In the street in the afternoon I met the non-addict father of a former patient from my rehab. I know she's doing well but he looked in poor shape. He's not looked after himself as well as she has and he's a decade younger than me.

My relationships – in both my general medical practice and my rehab – were personal, not academic. I loved the work and loved the people and I still do. My medical practice staff and I met up for a picnic lunch last weekend, eight years after we worked together. We do so twice a year.

I'm a people person, not an egg-head. I know the stuff – and I'm eager to learn more – but I love the people. In my work I need human experience as well as knowledge of the subject.

My counselling work speaks to my soul. For successful communication in that sphere I need to speak 'Addict'. It's a distinct language of its own, based on shared human experience rather than knowledge of the contents of textbooks.

Karen (ageless) was my medical practice secretary for its last seven years. Technically I employed her. But she ran me. I didn't have to think at all about the mechanics of running the practice. She did all that. She did the work she was good at and that left me free to do what I'm good at. Her practical experience enabled me to develop my 'spiritual' experience.

Chapter 21: Spirituality

The human spirit is alive inside all of us. It's up to us to find it.

When Dr Bob and Bill W expanded the Five Step programme of the Buchman Movement (Oxford Group) of evangelical Christians into the Twelve Step programme of Alcoholics Anonymous, they did so primarily to differentiate spirituality from religion.

After every mention of the word 'God', they inserted the underlined and italicised phrase *as you understand Him*. This enabled religious atheists or agnostics to join AA in order to treat their disease of the human spirit. There is even a chapter in the *Big Book* – story book – of AA that is headed, 'We Agnostics'. Clearly, they're on the inside.

A DVD, *Bill W*, tells the fascinating story of the early years of AA and the immense struggles that were surmounted. In appendix III of this book are the initial reviews of the *Big Book* in *The Journal of the American Medical Association* and *The American Journal of Nervous Mental Disorders*. They're well worth reading as examples of cynically dismissive vitriol.

On the other hand, John D Rockefeller, from whom the founding members of AA had hoped to gain financial support, said that he fully endorsed their ideas but money would destroy them.

This principle was followed in the UK when The House of Lords upheld the right of AA to refuse a large financial legacy when they said that the (written) Traditions include the statement that AA 'should be fully self-supporting, declining outside contributions'.

It has been said (in Native American sayings among others) that religion is for people who are afraid of going to hell; spirituality is for those who have already been there.

Yet the mere mention of the word 'God' in AA's Twelve Step programme leads many people to believe that it is a religious programme. This is what led me to write *A Book of Prayers for Atheists and Agnostics*. I wanted to show that the Twelve Step programme itself is my God (or Higher Power than self) and encourage others to do the same if they had difficulty with the word 'God' in the Twelve Steps.

Albert Ellis, the psychologist creator of Rational Emotive Behaviour Therapy (REBT) went so far as to write a *Little Book* as a deliberate parody on the *Big Book* of AA. Albert Ellis set up 'Drink Watchers' groups as a 'non-religious' alternative to AA meetings.

In London, Charles Vetter took over the defunct Western Fever Hospital and made it into a base for REBT ideas. It was hugely successful and Drink Watchers meetings became very popular. Members were encouraged to keep diaries of their drinking habits.

Charles Vetter's institution was financially supported by many firms from the City of London, particularly by ICI. His annual conference – that I attended one year in the old town hall in Kensington High Street – had David Ennals, the government Minister of Health, as its keynote speaker.

Then one day Charles Vetter changed his mind and supported the ideas of AA. His financial support was withdrawn and his institution collapsed and closed.

And Drink Watchers meetings did not survive.

But the ideas of REBT are still very much alive. They were originally taken up in the UK principally by Professor Windy Dryden of Goldsmith's College in London. And the NHS to this day recommends patients to keep drinking diaries.

And in Weight Watchers meetings slimmers tell each other their success stories.

In Alcoholics Anonymous meetings – and in offshoots in Narcotics Anonymous and similar 'Fellowships' for gamblers, cocaine addicts and many others – Twelve Step ideas are still flourishing.

Yet schisms occur. Food Addicts Anonymous make much more stringent requirements for abstinence than Overeaters Anonymous, which welcomes people with any form of eating disorder. People who have compulsive sexual behaviour can choose between Sexaholics Anonymous, Sex Addicts Anonymous and Sex and

Love Addicts Anonymous, each of which has its own particular stipulations for abstinence.

All this division and sub-division is healthy. AA itself is adamant that they make no rules. They stipulate that 'Even the Twelve Steps are merely suggested'.

Addicts of any kind will duck and dive and pontificate in many creative ways in order to avoid acknowledging that the problems go with their inside world rather than primarily with anything in the outside world.

SMART Recovery is merely one of the latest in a long line of therapeutic approaches that appeal to inner strength rather than the weakness that AA members acknowledge. Adherents to the SMART Recovery programme are discouraged from acknowledging any higher power than self. As with Drink Watchers and Weight Watchers, and people who follow the determinedly rational approach of REBT, these ideas are immensely popular. They fill up rehabs where commerce is the driving force, as opposed to focussing on getting patients well.

And Cognitive Behavioural Therapy (CBT) – on the principle of 'Think right and you will behave right' – remains as the dominant force in psychotherapy.

Whether any of the therapeutic approaches that lay claim to success in treating addicts (and they all do) actually achieve positive results depends upon their definitions of 'abstinence' and 'recovery'. Generally, in the counselling world, these goalposts can be shifted all over the park. But not in AA.

The Twelve Step programme continues as it began. It is a spiritual programme, looking at spiritual values such as hope, love, trust, honour, beauty, innocence and generosity while rejecting arrogance and grandiosity and what their members term 'self-will run riot'.

I've been there, done that and got the T-shirt. Like Charles Vetter, my experience led me to change my mind.

Percival (65) was an ardent worshipper, even though his wife reminded him that he forcefully disagreed with every point the vicar made in his sermons. He was also 'a director of five major companies', as he liked to remind us in group therapy sessions on frequent occasions. He totally rejected any idea that he might have a problem with alcohol. One weekend I got his wife and each of his four children to spell out to him their concerns over his repeated drunken bouts. He told them they were imagining things. He left the treatment centre and was blind drunk within the hour. His religious beliefs had not protected him from his spiritual illness any further than the bottom of the hill.

Chapter 22: Confusion

'Confused' often means 'used' something addictive.

Addicts frequently complain of being confused when they want to avoid facing up to reality. I see 'confused' as meaning 'used': they have used a mood-altering substance or process that affects their perceptions.

Desperately, they want to prove to themselves – and to other people – that black is white in their concepts and behaviour. They hope that something will change their feelings and solve their problems. What they discover is that their feelings, as a result of using a mood-altering substance or behaviour, are never quite as good as the very first remarkable time. And the problems get progressively worse.

So, as made clear in the *Big Book*, they blame other people, places and things for their plight.

Recently a play called *People, Places and Things* told the story of a young addict. It presented her parents in a poor light, in effect blaming them for the poor little thing's lonely descent into addictive behaviour. The rehab scenes were brutal and the programme notes were scathing about Twelve Step approaches, while supporting the ideas of SMART Recovery. And addicts loved the play. They flocked to it and told each other about it.

Of course they did. It fed into their sense of blame and self-pity, the primary feelings of all using, rather than recovering, addicts. Even members of various Anonymous Fellowships – and especially those who had relapsed – thought it was a wonderful play. It said what they wanted to say to their families. It mirrored the popular beliefs of therapists who say that addiction comes from abuse and abandonment.

My family didn't abandon me by sending me 'home' from India to England. Responsibly, they gave me the precious gift of education. They and my guardians didn't abuse me in any way. Verbally, I abused them repeatedly. My school was abusive, but no more to me than to other boys. But I didn't abuse any other boy. I'm proud of that. I've learned never to treat other people in the negative ways some of them behave towards me. That's an extremely valuable lesson.

I choose to be polite and respectful to others because I choose that behavioural principle. I do not want other people to have power over my behaviour. I do not believe that I should necessarily behave badly towards people who behave badly towards me. I don't want to behave inconsiderately and abusively at any time. Not nowadays.

I could never survive the abuse I get – from some addicts and some of their family members – in my counselling work if I do not remember how abusive I have been to people who tried to help me by getting me to change my ideas, principles and behaviour.

We addicts don't want to change. Nobody does, but addicts definitely don't. At all. We are *not* confused. Emphatically not. It's just that we want the whole world to change to our way of thinking and behaving. And we find it puzzling when they don't.

We can all see that in the dreaming of adolescents and in the conniving promises of politicians who groom them by saying what they most want to hear. We see it in teachers who manipulate school curricula – particularly in history – in order to put forward their own personal and political agenda. We see it in the whole apparatus of welfare systems and religions that sanctify the downtrodden and never ask how they came to be in that situation. At the extreme, we see it in terrorists taking people's lives on the fundamental basis of having a 'right' and even a 'duty' to do so. Beliefs are presented as facts. Hopes are seen as entitlements. Ethics and principles are discarded in favour of slogans. And violent behaviour is normalised. And gentle people – to all personal accounts – become apologists for tyranny.

Jo (25) is impressionable. So she should be at her age. Hopefully so am I at any age. This weekend she's in Glastonbury at the rock festival. She's with her own kind, just as I shall be with mine in Glyndebourne's opera house. But whereas I see her choice of music as a personal preference, she sees mine as elitist and therefore deplorable. (Interestingly, she is in favour of state sponsorship of the Arts whereas I am not. I believe opera is appreciated most when our painful experiences in life resonate with those on stage and when we understand theatrical metaphor. We don't need to attract young people to opera. They will grow into it.) In our respective political views, I see Jo as a misguided young idealist. She sees me as evil. As far as mood-altering drugs are concerned, she sees their use as a personal choice, whereas I see them as *destroying* choice because I've seen so many lives damaged by their use. It's difficult for me to be open-minded on this issue because of the sheer amount of my personal and professional experience.

Chapter 23: Politics

All life is politics. We can't avoid it. But we can avoid being dragged down by it.

I want our healthcare and welfare systems to work effectively, particularly for the people who most need them. These services therefore have to be based on sound ideas. (Appendix V lists my suggestions.)

But political and religious beliefs have no place in meetings of the Anonymous Fellowships. Members look at what *unites* them rather than divides them.

Addiction is a significant feature in many people's lives. As I mentioned at the very beginning of this book, about one in six of us (17% of the population) are addicts by nature. Each one of us – obviously with considerable overlap in addictive families – significantly affects the lives of five other people. That adds up to a lot of trouble.

But politicians are remarkably uninterested in doing anything more significant than debate the legalisation of cannabis.

Politicians themselves have the same incidence of addictive disease as the rest of the population. But journalists tend to expect them to be the guardians of public morality as well as purse.

I am very much a political animal, interested in political ideas. But nowadays I see too many contradictions – in policy and practice – to be comfortable as a member of any political party.

In any case, as an addict, I have too many behavioural skeletons in my historical cupboard – albeit from over 30 years ago – to feel that risking exposure and vilification in a political position is worthwhile. There may be many other people who feel the same. The end result could be that many people with more talent than mine may feel equally that public service has too many elephant traps.

A further problem is that career politicians rarely have outside experience of any great significance. Their lives are bounded by procedures, precedents and references back for further discussion, rather than by taking decisions for which they will be held personally and financially, as well as politically, responsible. And the end result of that is that we get the – largely unimaginative – politicians we deserve. Literally they don't know what they're talking about.

I know of no politician, apart from Lord Mancroft, who really does understand addictive disease and recovery. And Benjamin would acknowledge that he is more of an administrator than clinician. Even though I have treated members of both Houses of Parliament, and advised some of them on addiction problems in their families, this hasn't been translated into parliamentary proposals or public policies. I'm a guilty secret.

As with doctors and psychiatrists and many other professionals, politicians who get into behavioural difficulty tend to put their problems down to 'stress'. They forget that many people have similar stressors. But how each of us reacts to them – and experiences 'stress' – is entirely our own peculiarity.

Parliamentary politicians are rarely in government posts for more than a few years. They get rotated through various departments. They get lots of experience of parliamentary procedure but at the price of relatively shallow understanding of any particular subject, such as healthcare and welfare in general, let alone addiction in particular. They may be on parliamentary committees that specialise in particular subjects but even then they are mostly guided by the Civil Service. And those 'Sir Humphrey's (with acknowledgement to the brilliant *Yes Minister* TV series) are advised by 'experts'.

On the subject of treatment for addiction, I once gave evidence to the Parliamentary Sub-committee on Health and Social Services. A member commented that I appeared to want to turn the whole system upside-down. I agreed, saying that the current approach didn't work. My brief moment of potential political influence didn't last beyond that point.

The elephant in the room is nothing to do with falling into elephant traps or avoiding them. It's the obvious problem that nobody wants to talk about. In this respect the body politic is similar to family members anywhere. They would rather not acknowledge the existence of a problem they don't know how to deal with.

Addicts – at all levels of society – need to be confronted. Politicians don't like doing that. They would rather spend other people's money doing things that are supportive and obviously 'sensible', even when there is no evidence of the ideas and practical procedures working in practice.

They certainly don't like to be told by me that addiction problems are probably genetic in origin. They want them to be social. They believe – with scant evidence – that they can do something about social problems. But they know they can't change someone's genes. Well, not yet to any great extent.

To be told by me that they don't need to do so causes even more confusion. To be shown that, through brain plasticity, we can change our nature through consistent daily change in our behaviour is downright disturbing for them. It implies that politicians aren't needed. That's their worst nightmare. Also – with reason – they believe they can't trust addicts to maintain their own recovery.

But that doesn't mean they can't do anything at all. They – and family members and counsellors – have to get involved in the civil war inside each addict and separate the individual from the disease, supporting the individual with rehab facilities while confronting the disease with punitive consequences.

But politicians like to be liked. That's how they get elected. So the problem continues, with no political or social solution in sight.

For my part, I hope that I shall always be friendly towards anyone. But I am no friend of addictive disease. I do everything I can to confront it.

Michael Stewart, Lord Stewart of Fulham, (1906 – 1990) was my mother's brother and the first of my childhood guardians. After glittering educational success in Oxford, where he was also President of the Oxford Union (the debating society), he entered Parliament as a Labour MP and rose to become Foreign Secretary, with John Foster Dulles as his American opposite number in the State Department. My uncle was a heavy smoker and he died, painfully, of cancer of the oesophagus. **Sir Harold Jeffreys (1891 – 1981)** was married to my mother's cousin. They were equally brilliant academics at Cambridge. He was a heavy smoker but he didn't die of it. Intellects, such as his and my uncle's, are no protectors against addiction. Genes are sometimes protective, as they appear to have been in Sir Harold's case.

Chapter 24: Despair

The gift of desperation is when we've had enough pain from trying to prove that black is white.

AA members refer to 'the gift of desperation' getting them into recovery. They recognised they could not go on as they were. The widespread consequences of their addictive behaviour had mounted up. Their personal and professional relationships had often disintegrated. In that situation in my own life, I looked around for my friends and found they weren't there.

During the short time I was admitted to a mental nursing home, I had no visitors whatever. Family members, personal friends and professional colleagues had had more than enough of me. Thinking back to those days now, decades later, I feel just a bit sorry for myself. I was still in full-time work, paying my way and educating my children. In that limited sense I was a responsible member of society. And I was still creative in looking for new ideas. In a blank room on my own I certainly needed some. I had to reflect on the demonstrable fact that nobody else felt sorry for me.

There was no point in re-visiting ideas I had had before. They had brought me to this spiritual dead-end. But where could I go? I didn't know. I despaired.

If I had not been totally mad before going into the mental nursing home, I was certainly going that way in an environment of sensory deprivation. I had nothing to do or look at or read, nothing to listen to, nobody to talk to. I was as isolated as a convict in solitary confinement even though I was there voluntarily because I wanted my wife back. Somehow.

My childhood fear had been of being on my own. Yet my reality at that time was far from that. Even though my parents and my brother were in India – and our only contact for four years was by weekly letter – I was well cared for by my guardians and I was surrounded by other boys at school. My friends in the choir and in the Boy Scout troop were real friends, several of whom I still see today.

I was far from lonely at the time of our shared childhoods. Nor am

I lonely today. I have lots of personal friends. But in the blank room of the mental nursing home I was very lonely indeed, in the deepest pit of despair. I recognised that, if I stayed where I was, I would die by my own hand if no other.

So I left (and, incidentally, never heard from the psychiatrist who had put me there and whose fees had been paid by my private medical insurance company for those three days, even though he made no contact with me then or since.)

I told Meg that she could have the children and the house and half my income for the rest of my life but she couldn't have me at the price I was paying at that time. She said that she had been thinking of coming back… So we worked things out and got back together. I certainly didn't want to go through that experience of utter loneliness and despair again.

Since that time – or soon after – my closest confidants have been people in the Anonymous Fellowships – and I have even got used to that term because I can think of no better one to describe our mutual support.

I know some of them personally because they have been patients of mine in my rehab. But the only things I know about most of the others are their first names and their addiction stories. Yet I know them better than I know my brother. I see them every week. Mostly, I don't know where they live or what they do, whether they're single or married. I often do know if they come from the gay, lesbian, bisexual and intersex community because they tend to talk about it. They find acceptance in the Fellowships a refreshing contrast to the prejudice they often still find elsewhere.

I myself am very happy to be anonymous. My life is often too public for my personal comfort. I like what is described in the *Big Book* as 'the fraternity of strangers'. In that company I counter my denial – I see my own addictive nature reflected in the mirror of theirs – and I have no sense of inner loneliness and despair at all.

Lance (44) was referred to me by a consultant psychiatrist who despaired of him and his anorexia. I doubt the referral was an act of friendship to Lance or to me. Certainly I have never heard from that specialist again. I think he wanted to teach me a lesson that I should not take on the care of 'real' patients.

I put Lance into my rehab and he did very well. He liked the company. When I told him I thought he was gay, he was very upset. That was the last thing he wanted on top of having to accept his addictive nature. But he did. Today – nearly 20 years later – he lives happily with his boyfriend and they run a successful business together. I see him regularly in Fellowship meetings. He's in very good physical, mental, emotional and spiritual shape. He has no reason whatever to despair and absolutely no need of medical supervision or psychiatry. He gets on with his life.

Chapter 25: New Hope

When we see people like us getting well we know we're on the right track.

I have hope. Lots of it. I've been in a professional and personal abyss and emerged on the other side. I've been widowed and bankrupted but here I am, married to Pat and earning my living through my outpatient rehab services. I've lived through frightening political circumstances and I'm sure I have the resilience to do so again. Also – and most significantly – I've accepted my addictive nature and I do the things I need to do each day to keep it in remission. I have absolutely no reason to despair and every reason to have hope.

My professional work involves me giving a sense of hope to others. I'm not simply providing information and sensible advice. That never turned me round on my addictive path. My purpose in telling so much of my own story in this book is to show that abstinence from all mood-altering substances and processes, and working the Twelve Step programme every day of my life, has given me peace of mind and great happiness. Despite dreadful past events and significant fears for the future, I walk with a light step and with my head held high.

Pat and I have been to four operas recently. This is the time of year when the English countryside is at its most beautiful best. Glyndebourne is in the Sussex downs, Longborough Opera is in the Cotswold hills. We seeped ourselves in beauty, on-stage and off.

Back in the 'real world', I've attended an addiction conference in London. That experience was equally inspiring. Hearing Benjamin Mancroft speak knowledgeably and sensitively was a privilege and pleasure. Hearing Shane Varcoe, a Demand Reduction Education and Advocacy Specialist I'd never heard before, was a delight. Finding a kindred spirit in the wilderness of talks about strategic policy, professional accreditation and financial management was very refreshing.

Shane believes in minimising harm by maximising prevention. To this aim he told me that decriminalisation of drugs is a step towards legalisation. I learned from him.

I didn't need Mindfulness meditation or yoga or massage or music therapy, all of which were demonstrated in the conference. I need someone with the mind and clinical experience to challenge my ideas. And I got it from Shane.

And that is exactly what newcomers to the Anonymous Fellowships and new patients in a rehab most need. They need to be *inspired* rather than patronised. They need to be shown that there is a tried and trusted way through their confusion and despair. They need to be given *hope*.

This doesn't need an army of professionals. It can be provided by one person with a warm heart and clear mind to go with his or her vital personal experience.

I don't judge individuals on their 'clean time' – years, months or days – of abstinence. Nor do I judge counsellors on their professional qualifications. I want to see the glint in the eye and sense the enthusiasm. And I want to hear that people have got their own lives in order despite difficult challenges. I want evidence that what people are talking about works in practice for them. I don't want to hear them talk about honesty, open-mindedness and willingness – the H-O-W of recovery. I want to witness it in every aspect of their lives.

Of course that's a tall order. It has to be. Addiction is the major killer, not only directly through suicide and overdoses and other tragic consequences but indirectly via substances and processes leading to cancer, heart disease, diabetes, mania and other physical and mental illnesses. Counsellors have to be warm-hearted and strong-minded. Otherwise they have nothing of value to offer. And they would not be in a position to give hope to anyone.

Rachael (47) works in the addiction field. She has financial success because she has personal charm and because she tells her patients what they want to hear. The story won't end happily for them. Or for her.

Chapter 26: Failure

We should be proud of our failures. At least we tried.
Now we can learn better ways.

I've had many glorious failures.

My first hope was to be a professional musician. I failed.

Later on, in addition to being a doctor, I tried politics. I failed.

And farming. I failed again.

I've written seven novels. No agent or publisher has picked them up. Yet.

I've written the lyrics for a musical but I lack the skill to write the music.

There is nothing left of my medical practice or rehab or extended care facilities. The buildings have been changed out of recognition or destroyed by fire. Deliberately.

To be sure, I've had many failures and I anticipate I'll have many more. And there may be more destruction.

So what? I've lived and loved, had ideas and created. And I still do all of that.

I do not acknowledge any of the events in my life as a 'success' or 'failure'. As with Rudyard Kipling in his poem *If*, I don't acknowledge those imposters. I've had a fabulous journey and I haven't yet arrived at the destination. I don't even know where it is, other than in spiritual terms. My life is mine. I want to be me.

But I do know that there's only one thing I want to say to my Creator or to the evolutionary Blind Watchmaker: "Thank you!".

I do not pepper my prose with exclamation marks or punctuate my writing with emoticons. I have real relationships and real feelings. My energy and enthusiasm are as bright and boundless as ever. I'm younger in spirit than many people less than half my natal age.

My attitudes and activities are gifts that come directly from daily working of the Twelve Step programme and putting into practice the well-known fragment of Reinhold Neuberger's Serenity Prayer:

'God grant me the serenity
To accept the things I cannot change,
Courage to change the things I can
And the wisdom to know the difference.'

That's what I believe. Because it works for me. If other people want what I've got in my human spirit, that's fine. If they don't, that's also fine. It's their choice. I hope they find happy and fulfilling lives in their own ways.

Of course I recognise that I've had a privileged upbringing and education and wonderful professional opportunities. I've been very fortunate in many ways. Most of all I've benefitted from learning to do things that benefit me and not do things that harm me. Yes, that's been difficult at times but the outcome is fabulous.

David (50ish) is a creative artist, a magnificent one. He brings a lot of happiness to other people's lives. But he had little in his own. Like many others in his profession, he was depressed. He 'treated' this 'depression' with alcohol and other artificial 'help', such as so-called 'antidepressants'. As I see it, he was born with an addictive nature, developed a sense of inner emptiness, and stuck out his antennae in trying to make sense of the crazy surroundings in his childhood. This led to him becoming highly creative. That's the way round it is: not that creative people become addicts but that addicts become creative. Nowadays David doesn't see his life as being a success or a failure but, as many addicts say, he's glad to be an addict because he's benefitted so much – in many areas of life – from working the Twelve Step programme.

Chapter 27: Humility

False humility is creepy. The genuine article is gentle and warm.

If we say we're humble, or even think we are, we aren't. Fortunately, every one of the Twelve Steps is an exercise in humility.

I. We admitted we were powerless over alcohol (or any addiction), that our lives had become unmanageable.
My various addictive behaviours drove me forward in the arrogant belief that I could do whatever I wanted but not have to face the consequences.

II. Came to believe that a Power greater than ourselves could restore us to sanity.
My life was a mess. I created that mess. To believe otherwise – against all the evidence – was madness.

III. Made a decision to turn our will and our lives over to the care of God _as we understood Him._
If I'm sufficiently clear on Steps I and II this Step is obvious. Turning my life over to a higher power than self is easy. I could be struck down by fate at any time. Turning over my will is another matter altogether. I'm very determined and strong-willed. That's why it took me until the age of 47 to get into recovery.

IV. Made a searching and fearless moral inventory of ourselves.
This Step is straightforward. I know what I've done. Doing this Step thoroughly – in bullet points rather than in a long-winded self-serving essay – has beneficial knock-on effects on Steps VI and VIII.

V. Admitted to God, to ourselves and to another human being the exact nature of our wrongs.
Whatever higher power I choose to have, I assume that my guilty secrets are already known. Telling someone else about them is tricky. But I can't afford to be bashful, let alone secretive, if I want to get well and stay well.

VI. Were entirely ready to have God remove all these defects of character.

This Step is necessary because Step VII is so huge.

VII. Humbly asked Him to remove our shortcomings.

Humbly? I don't do 'humble'. I do things my way, as the song says.

Asked? I don't ask; I tell.

God? Who?

To remove? Do something?

My. For me?

Defects of character? Yes please. Otherwise I'll go round the loop again. I've had enough pain.

VIII. Made a list of all persons we had harmed, and became willing to make amends to them all.

Addicts like to put their own names top of the list. Compulsive helpers tend to believe they've harmed everyone they've ever met. The truth is probably closer to being the other way round.

IX. Made direct amends to such people wherever possible, except when to do so would injure them or others.

Living amends – changing our behaviour – are most appropriate to those people who are closest to us. They've heard us say sorry 1,000 times so that word is no longer viable currency. Face-to-face amends are very difficult but that's why the 'Promises' of recovery (specified in Chapter 28) are specifically attached to Step IX in the *Big Book*. They do not fall out of the sky, like heavenly manna, simply as a result of going to Fellowship meetings.

X. Continued to take personal inventory and when we were wrong promptly admitted it.

This is another tricky Step but it has to be done if recovery is to be maintained.

XI. Sought through prayer and meditation to improve our conscious contact with God *as we understood Him,* praying only for knowledge of His will for us and the power to carry that out.

The mode of prayer and meditation are personal choices. The word 'only' in the second part of this Step is crucial. For prayers to be effective in changing addictive behaviour, they need to be a lot more than shopping lists.

XII. Having had a spiritual awakening as the result of these steps, we tried to carry this message to alcoholics and to practice these principles in all our affairs.

Carrying the message does not mean that it will be heard and accepted. *Being* the message – and showing acceptance and gratitude – is more likely to be effective. Practising (with the English spelling of the verb) the principles of honesty, open-mindedness and willingness in everything we do is another tricky one, applying as much to our dealings with the Inland Revenue as to anything else.

Cynics often say that the concept of addictive disease and its treatment with the Twelve Step programme are cop-outs. I doubt they've ever contemplated doing Steps V and IX themselves. My own continuing journey through the Steps has been the hardest challenge I have ever faced.

I've been through training – in National Service – as a junior army officer in the Royal Signals, before I ever thought of becoming a doctor. Putting up telegraph lines on the North Yorkshire moors for three days and two nights in the snow wasn't a cake-walk.

Being the junior hospital doctor on the heart ward – at the time when cardiac resuscitation techniques were just coming in – was very tough. I had to live in the hospital, despite having a wife and child, and I was exhausted physically and emotionally when over 100 people died under my hands in my six month stint.

And I've been to British private boarding school (on a Local Authority financial grant). Anyone who can survive that experience – typified at that time by the book *Tom Brown's School Days* – can survive anything.

Working the Twelve Step programme has been harder than any of that. It has no time limit. But taking life one day at a time, as suggested in the *Big Book,* makes the challenge easier to meet.

I worked right through the Steps systematically with Fellowship sponsors – guides (one for my primary addictions and one for my compulsive helping) who have walked the same path before me. (I called my addiction sponsor just now and I see my own sponsees once a week.) I use 'the maintenance Steps' – X, XI and XII – every day. I say my prayers in the shower. I'm never going to forget to have a shower so I always remember to say my prayers, my psychological reminders on how I want to behave.

One way or another, I get myself into a routine. I go to three Fellowship meetings every week and I do a 'chair' (starting off the meeting with my own account of how my life used to be, what happened to turn me round, and how my life is now) whenever I am asked. I always say "Yes" before I ask where and when. Little habits – disciplines, professional behaviours – like this keep my recovery, such as it is, ticking over.

My anonymity as a Fellowship member is inevitably blown in this book. It has to be if I am to demonstrate that I know my subject. I've tried any number of other ways of controlling my addictive behaviour. They didn't work. So now I simply accept that I'm an addict by nature.

But there are two risks in squandering my anonymity. First, I might get carried away with my own significance and relapse. Second, my relapse would undo all the good that I am trying to do in this book. It would bring discredit to the Fellowship principles I describe. I have no doubt – and my own Fellowship sponsor would insist – that I am merely an addict, one among many others, doing my best to stay in recovery one day at a time and doing whatever I can to encourage other addicts to get into recovery. I am not a guru. God forbid.

Felicity (28) is a young mother. She therefore really does know everything about everything. Her chances of getting into long-term recovery are not good. It has to be her number one priority – even before looking after her baby. There is a sad – and frightening – saying in the Fellowships that we shall lose anything we put ahead of working our recovery programme. I hope she wises up – and becomes sufficiently humble to listen to others – before her husband leaves or the Social Services take away her baby.

Chapter 28: Rewards

The rewards of recovery are fabulous: beyond all hopes.

As I said in Chapter 27, 'The Promises' of recovery come from working Step IX. They don't come any other way. Reading them or reciting them at the end of Fellowship meetings doesn't deliver the goods. As with anything else of value in life, they have to be worked for. Here they are:

'If we are painstaking about this phase of our development, we will be amazed before we are half way through. We are going to know a new freedom and a new happiness. We will not regret the past nor wish to shut the door on it. We will comprehend the word serenity and we will know peace. No matter how far down the scale we have gone, we will see how our experience can benefit others. That feeling of uselessness and self-pity will disappear. We will lose interest in selfish things and gain interest in our fellows. Self-seeking will slip away. Our whole attitude and outlook upon life will change. Fear of people and of economic insecurity will leave us. We will intuitively know how to handle situations which used to baffle us. We will suddenly realise that God is doing for us what we could not do for ourselves.'

Then there's the catch that comes next:

'Are these extravagant promises? We think not. They are being fulfilled among us – sometimes quickly, sometimes slowly. They will always materialise if we *work* for them.'

Yes. That's the catch: if we want all these promises to come true in our lives, we have to do the footwork that makes it likely they will come true. Otherwise these spiritual promises would be no more valid than the promises of politicians eager to get – buy – votes.

So have they come true for me? Let me check...

'If we are painstaking about this phase of our development, we will be amazed before we are half way through.'

Yes. I have worked painstakingly on Step IX. Living amends – by changing my actions – have been straightforward. Direct amends have been more challenging because many of the people to whom I wished to make amends – including my wife, Meg – are dead. So I sat on my own in my office and imagined that each one of those people, in turn, was with me. I spoke out loud to them. When it came to Meg, I had to come back the next day and do it again. I felt I hadn't gone deep enough. And then I did it again on a third day until I felt I really had given this Step my best shot.

'We are going to know a new freedom and a new happiness.' Yes. I did feel free. I'm not sure I felt happy – except that my behaviour in those relationships doesn't haunt me any more.

'We will not regret the past nor wish to shut the door on it.' Yes. The past is past. The best I can say about much of my childhood is that it's over. But I learned very valuable lessons from it.

'We will comprehend the word serenity and we will know peace.' Yes. I understand serenity as peace of mind in spite of unsolved problems.

'No matter how far down the scale we have gone, we will see how our experience can benefit others.'

Yes. I do that in my professional work, although that doesn't count. I get paid for it and I'm not anonymous. But I also do it by sharing my thoughts and feelings in Fellowship meetings and by working systematically through all of the Steps with my sponsees. That does count.

'That feeling of uselessness and self-pity will disappear.'

Yes it's gone. Certainly the self-pity. I find that particular behaviour singularly unattractive.

'We will lose interest in selfish things and gain interest in our fellows.'

Yes. I'm much more interested in other people's personal welfare than I used to be, even as a doctor. I would like people to be as happy as I am. I'm absolutely not a 'happy-clappy' God-botherer. I'm just very privileged in finding an emotional therapeutic programme that works for me. I'm happy to talk about the Twelve Step programme if people want me to. But I don't knock on doors or walk around with a beatific smile. And I know how to growl if I want to in appropriate circumstances.

'Self-seeking will slip away.'

Yes. I'm content to own nothing and be nothing other than myself. I'm not the head of anything and I'm not looking for anything other than appreciation of my professional work and the opportunity to put my ideas forward. And I accept that I have to earn all that.

'Our whole attitude and outlook upon life will change.'

I've always enjoyed challenges. I like seeing where a new idea or way of doing things might lead. But nowadays I'm much better at taking life as it comes.

'Fear of people and of economic insecurity will leave us.'

I've been attacked, with people wanting to destroy my ideas as well as my property. (I've twice been on the receiving end of arson and several times had people try to put me out of business. But my ideas go with me and I've got plenty more where the last lot came from.) I'm still up and running and there's a great deal more I want to do in my life before I pop my clogs.

'We will intuitively know how to handle situations which used to baffle us.'

Yes. I no longer have any cravings to use mood-altering substances and processes. My mind is clear. I do what I believe is good for me – being kind to other people and supportive of them within the boundary of compulsive helping.

'We will suddenly realise that God is doing for us what we could not do for ourselves.'

Yes. I've come through dreadful experiences. Sometimes – such as when Meg died and I was stuck in the old people's home with nothing material or professional and no prospect of getting anything – I just put one foot in front of another. I worked Steps X, XI and XII each day. And here I am now, as happy and creative as I've ever been. My recovery – through working the Twelve Step programme – has given me a life prized above rubies.

I've lost many things but there's nothing that I've given up voluntarily – in the course of my recovery – that I value. I should be so fortunate to be able to enjoy the life I have now.

Silly men and women (adults chronologically but not spiritually) have all the toys – houses, cars, trinkets, relationships on the side, you name it – they set their hearts on. And they're poisoned by that lifestyle and personal philosophy. Happiness cannot be bought or demanded. Even so, in simple material terms, I agree with those who say 'I've been rich and I've been poor. Rich is better!'.

Chapter 29: Challenges

Who ever said life would be easy?

Setting up my rehab was the greatest challenge of my professional life. I had never been in rehab myself and it was only two years since I attended that first meeting in the Red Cross centre. That was not the strongest starting position I could have had.

I got the idea of creating a rehab when I referred a medical practice patient of mine to the Charter Clinic in Chelsea. I had been called to see him by his wife. There he was, a distinguished professional, hopelessly drunk, naked and face down in the entrance hall of his home in the middle of the day. I called one of the patients I had met in that first meeting in the Red Cross centre and he recommended this clinic. I visited this new patient every evening in the Charter Clinic, after I had finished work in my medical practice, for the six weeks he was there. The staff – apart from the duty nurse and night watchman – had gone home. I learned from the patients.

I could not have asked for better training. They told me their personal experience of the disastrous consequences of believing sensible drinking would be a far more secure position than abstinence. They had tried it many times and it hadn't worked. When I enquired about their childhoods, their family lives and their work situations, they told me that each of their situations was unique except for addiction of one kind or another in previous generations of their families. When I said they appeared to have every material thing anyone would ever wish for in life, they agreed.

I learned from them about the Twelve Step approach that they themselves were learning during the day.

They suggested that I would learn more if I were to join them as a patient. I excused myself by saying that I wasn't aware that I had an addiction problem. Nor was there one in my family, as far as I knew.

I checked this with my parents. My father said that his father drank a bit. – I learned later that he rarely did anything else. – And my mother said, "We used to find the bottles behind the Jane Austen books". I've got my grandmother's books now, as reminders that alcoholism can affect distinguished headmistresses just as much as anyone else.

I spoke to Bruce Lloyd, the head counsellor at the Charter Clinic. He and his wife, Bobby, who was the head counsellor at the North London Charter Clinic, came round to my medical practice one evening and talked to me about addictive disease and recovery for a couple of hours. I was spellbound. And surprised that I had never learned about this in three years at Cambridge University and another three years at The Middlesex Hospital in London. I had had the best medical education in the UK and had been taught *not one lesson* on addiction as such, rather than on what to do about its medical consequences.

Bruce and Bobby suggested I might go to Hazelden, the rehab in Minnesota where there was a 'professionals in residence' programme.

So I did. I had anticipated that I would be talking to the staff. Ha! They knew better. I slept in a visitor's room but during each day, they opened the door to one of the rehab units, ushered me in and closed the door. Again I learned from the patients. I went to their lectures and attended their group therapy sessions. I had my meals with them and I spoke to them hour after hour. In those two weeks I got to know them – and their addiction problems – very well indeed.

And I felt completely at home. They were 'my people' in a way I had never experienced previously at any time in my life. I remember them clearly 34 years later. Among others, there was a New York stock-broker, a Chicago cop, a Kentucky horse thief and an insurance agent from Maine, to whom the Kentucky man said, "I've seen a barn burning and a horse whipping but I've never seen anything quite as strange as you".

Oh yes. Oh yes. These were my people. When I left, they gave me a copy of *The Twelve Steps and Twelve Traditions*. (I already had a *Big Book*.) They had bought it for me and each of them signed it. I've still got it.

So, on my return to London, still only a few weeks into my own recovery from using mood-altering substances and processes, I told Meg that I wanted to set up a rehab. Long-sufferingly, she knew that there would be no stopping me in one of my enthusiasms. But she shared it when she came with me – twice – on the Hazelden family programme. In a further three visits to Hazelden I saw the extended care facility for particularly challenging patients, including the Chicago cop, the halfway house and the alumni centre. I knew that I would want to provide similar facilities and services. After all, Hazelden had started as Hazel's den – at the bottom of her garden – where her own long-suffering spouse had allowed her to indulge her passion in looking after a handful of alcoholics.

At the time I was there, Hazelden had something like 120 patients and a vast number of staff, with more than 400 of them working in the world-renowned publications department. (Today Hazelden works alongside the Betty Ford Centre in running 17 sites across America.)

I asked Harold Conlow, the treatment director – who always kept a *Big Book* on his desk – what my main problems would be likely to be. I anticipated that he would say cocaine or violence. But he said, "In the short term your problems are going to be staff. And – in the long term – your problems are going to be staff".

He was right.

But first I had to get some money and find a building. So I set up a charity. Through my private medical practice, I knew many members of the Great and the Good. Our trustees were the greatest and the goodest... and after a year we had raised not a penny. The medical charities weren't interested in helping a private doctor, even one who said he would take no income from the rehab. The drug companies weren't interested in helping an abstinence-based programme that didn't use medicinal drugs other than for short term detox. And people in general couldn't see how I would be able to run my medical practice – in order to earn my living – and the rehab at the same time.

So I had no choice but to borrow the money myself, by remortgaging everything we had, and buying a building in East Kent where we already had our weekend cottage and near where my parents lived in Canterbury. We spent as much on altering the building as we had in buying it. So we got what we wanted. The building already had planning permission for a nursing home so that was one hurdle we didn't have to jump.

But where would we find our staff and how would we train them?

Our Trust very kindly said they would provide the money to take my future staff for training in Hazelden. I took their letter to my bank, borrowed the necessary money for the training and travel, and scratched around the Fellowships to see if anyone wanted to do counselling work. Some did. And they knew others. And they knew counsellors who wanted to move from their present positions in one or other of the very few rehabs that existed at that time. A local family doctor said he would provide medical cover and a specialist, who happened to be a member of AA, said she would provide consultant cover.

So, with high hopes and eager anticipation, 16 of us trooped off to Hazelden. My staff learned the mechanics – paperwork largely – involved in running a rehab, while I spent time with senior staff. In the second week I visited the Betty Ford Centre in California and Patrick Carnes, the foremost expert in treating sex and love addiction, in Golden Valley in Minnesota. They were exciting times.

What followed was not great. I didn't see my rehab director for three months. He said he was looking for patients. He never found any. So I let him go. The family counsellor sat in his office, expecting me – magically – to find patients for him. He saw none in three months so I let him go as well. The family doctor resigned. He said his wife didn't want him to work with addicts. The wife of the assistant director went off with one of the other counsellors, leaving behind a very angry husband. Another counsellor was admitted to hospital in a psychiatric emergency.

Then the Trust told me they could not give me the money after all. Trust law forbids them to promise money they had not already raised. When I told that to my bank they closed my accounts, not only on the rehab but also on my medical practice.

But I had friends. The pathology laboratory said that I could let their charges – in my medical practice and in the rehab – mount up until I could afford to pay them. Local traders in East Kent said the same. My rich Arab patients – whom many people assumed would bail me out – did no such thing. I didn't ask them or anyone else. Rich people remain rich by hanging on to their money, although the chairman of our Trust gave me a substantial donation to fund outcome studies.

I got myself into the mess. It was up to me to get out of it. As it happened, property prices were going up and – after a year – I was able to re-mortgage and settle all my trading debts.

At the very beginning we had a dry run for two weeks – with dummy patients collected from the Fellowships – and then I sent in four patients from my medical practice, including one with anorexia – the first patient in the UK with an eating disorder to be treated in an addiction rehab. Subsequently we treated the first gambler and the first sex and love addict. We tried to treat the first nicotine addict as a day patient but he ran off immediately. Even today, when nicotine addiction has the worst general medical consequences of all addictions (anorexia has the highest mortality rate) it is exceedingly difficult to get nicotine addicts to see themselves as *addicts* rather than merely as cigarette smokers. Nicotine Anonymous rarely survives more than a few months when it is tried in the UK.

But that was the least of my professional problems. In the next seven weeks we had no new patients. I had no choice but to take in some freebies, just to keep the place going. The arrangement was that I would treat them without charge but then they would pay me £10 a week out of their dole money or earnings for one year. I took in fifty freebies, one after another. I once received one £10 note.

People who know nothing whatever about the complexities of setting up and running a rehab, are full of bright ideas that don't work in practice. I know they don't. I've tried them.

In our courtyard I had brick inlays of small circles. Smokers had to stand inside one of those circles in isolation, unable to make their behaviour into a social occasion. I once tried to make the rehab non-smoking but I lost two counsellors and four patients immediately. I didn't take the counsellors back onto the staff because I cannot see how they could work with patients' feelings while suppressing their own. But I had to relax my prohibition for patients or go out of business. The disease won that particular battle. It won another when I discovered years later that some of my remaining counselling staff had continued to smoke. But I've won many other battles against addictive disease – temporarily I know: we can never afford to be complacent in recovery – so I don't complain.

I didn't complain in later years when two of my counselling directors – one after another – left my employment in order to set up a rival organisation. If that's what they want to do, good luck to them. I don't own my staff or my patients.

And I didn't complain when I was taken to court by a man I had hoped to employ to do PR work for me. I had to withdraw the offer when I was told by one of my patients that he was his supplier of cocaine. When I telephoned him to say that, he asked that I should talk to him in person. So I went round to his office, only to discover that it was open-plan. I wrote out – on a crossed-out private prescription, 'I can't take you on because of your own drug use'. He took me to court to find out the name of my informant. I'm sure he knew who it was but I wasn't going to betray a medical confidence. It would close my rehab if I were to do so. I said exactly that to the magistrate. He told me that legal requirements override medical confidentiality and that I would be in contempt of court – with the risk of a custodial sentence until I had purged my contempt – if I did not disclose the name. I was given two weeks to think it over. I replied immediately that I would not divulge the name at any time. I was still given two weeks to ponder the seriousness of my legal position. During that two weeks the man withdrew the case. I breathed again.

I spoke to Max Glatt, the psychiatrist who set up the addiction unit in Wormwood Scrubs prison and another in Warlingham Park prison, about this and about my various other problems, including my irritation with the press for repeatedly printing the opposite of what I had said.

He paused. He looked at me kindly and with understanding...

And I realised that I had been self-pitying in a conversation with a refugee German Jew.

Ted (40) told me that his grandmother had left him a lovely house in the country. He was sure it would make a wonderful rehab. He asked for my advice. I said – I hope not unkindly – that there are hundreds of houses that would make great rehabs but he would have to start with getting the right ideas in place, and then the right staff, before he thought about buildings.

Chapter 30: Families

Coming from an addictive family is hard. Bringing up an Addictive family is harder.

In my rehab we found there were only two factors that significantly influenced outcome:

1. Dealing with *all* addictive outlets, as revealed on my questionnaires (see the full list in Appendix II) and in particular, giving up smoking.
2. Family members attending our family group sessions.

My lectures (some of them can be seen on YouTube) and my psychodrama sessions led to no demonstrable benefit in relapse prevention. Patients and their families appreciated them - mostly - but they didn't help. That was not the information I wanted to hear from my research department but that's too bad. I continued to do them because they bonded patients together. This was vital in preparing them for future attendance in Fellowship meetings. Mutual help is what works. When A reaches out to help B, it is A - the helper - who gets better. B - the recipient - may or may not.

Meg trained first as a physiotherapist, then as a secretary, then as a teacher (She had a BEd degree in education), then as a medical laboratory scientist (to help me in my private medical practice) and finally as a Rogerian person-centred counsellor. (She commented that every change of plan in my life involved her in doing more work.) That was sadly true. She hated the lab work but loved the counselling she did with families.

And that had significant beneficial results.

Whereas previous family counsellors would get five or six family members coming to their groups on a Sunday morning, Meg regularly attracted 30. She knew how to love people and they loved her. Over 1,000 people - many of them family members she had helped - attended her memorial service.

She and I expanded the weekly family group into a whole range of family services:

- Family groups in London during the week as well as in Kent at the weekends.
- Conjoint sessions, in London and Kent, with a patient and his or her family.
- Intervention sessions with potential new patients who were reluctant to accept they had addiction problems.
- A lecture I gave every Sunday morning in Kent to all the patients and their families, sometimes totalling over 100.
- A weekly family therapy group run by Meg in London.
- A one-week residential workshop in London (where we had 24 beds in our follow-on and outpatient facility) for family members. I contributed to that but it was primarily run by Meg, once every two or three months.

Incidentally, Meg also took no income from our addiction work. We didn't want to run a business. Working with patients and their families is what we wanted to do. We aimed to provide services that we ourselves had not received – at all – when we asked for help initially for our own family.

Our children were grown up by the time we were doing all this work. But Meg regretted, to the day of her death, that she had not spent more time with our children when they were young. Even though Meg knew a stay-at-home mother of five addicts, she was still sad that she had worked with me when the children were young. I have to live with that. Certainly, as an addict, I was very self-centred in those days. Maybe I still am. It's difficult to judge ourselves.

Judging other people's behaviour is only too easy. To make a judgement, an assessment on whether someone's action is sensible or otherwise, is fair enough. But to be judgemental, dismissing the person, is not. Politicians tend to do a lot of that. My uncle never did. A Conservative opponent once said that it was always a pleasure to hear him speak. My rabidly left-wing aunt said he had to do something to make the Tories hate him. He never did. He has been an immense influence upon me.

Meg was like that. She accepted people as they are but gently challenged their ideas. Senior partners of legal firms, accountants, doctors, housewives, all would listen to her and learn from her in the family groups. Yet she described herself as being "here to guide the traffic".

One thing we both did was to try to help patients and their families to do things that *worked*. Time and again families are keen to know precisely what particular illegal drugs look like and what their street names are. We asked them why on earth they would want to know. Meg herself didn't know any of that stuff. She didn't need to. She and I actively discouraged families from trying to find out more about drugs as such. Rather than searching children's rooms for substances, they would learn more about what was going on by watching their children's behaviour, their relationships and their school achievements. If they saw a progressive decline in standards, they would know there's an addict in the home. Then they should call us. We understand their concerns because we've had them. But we know what works and what doesn't. Doctors, and even psychiatrists, would sometimes not know how to intervene kindly and persuasively unless they themselves had a Twelve Step background.

Let me be absolutely clear on this: giving information has very little benefit. It leads only to requests for even more information. Families can become just as obsessed as addicts. And their lives can become just as unbalanced. I write and talk about my personal life and social activities because I've got a real life. I do things I enjoy. I don't do things that upset my peace of mind. I can look at social and political ideas and actions and be appropriately concerned for the future. But I can still do my counselling work, write my books and sleep at night. When family members become obsessed over a loved one's behaviour, they sometimes can't function. Their lives fall to pieces in exactly the same way that the lives of active addicts fall to pieces. This does not encourage others to follow their actions.

I do not underestimate the difficult decisions family members may have to take. Yesterday I was asked how to intervene in a young girl's anorexia. The difficulty was that her school work and her social behaviour is perfect. Her family had been trying to control her food intake. They tried pleading with her. On a weekend break from boarding school they sat with her at mealtimes. They listened to her talking about calories, diets, health foods and vitamins. They said they understood her need for exercise but felt what she had been doing was perhaps a bit excessive.

My suggestion was that they should write to the school doctor, detailing their precise concerns. That will put the fear of God into the doctor. He will need to take clinical action – for fear of being clobbered in the courts and by the General Medical Council if the worst happens – while the parents, if they can bring themselves to do so, go to the cinema.

There's yet another story in today's newspapers on the 'failures' of a particular private psychiatric hospital. The expectation is that they should cure illness, educate in order to prevent relapse and, in particular, reduce to zero any risk of self-harm or suicide. That can't be done.

So, out of self-protection, doctors prescribe, prescribe and prescribe so they can say to the courts and coroners that they did all they could and followed the actions of their professional peers. That is clinical inertia; absolutely deadly clinical inertia. The doctor is covered but the patient is dead, spiritually if not physically.

That is precisely why I do the work I do. I don't want a contented clinical life, doing what I was trained to do and keeping in line. I want to find out whatever I can about other ways of helping patients with their compulsive behaviour that leads to devastating consequences.

But first I have to gain the trust of family members by telling them the truth: *you* didn't cause this problem, *you* don't contribute to it getting worse and *you* can't cure it.

They will hear exactly that same message in AlAnon family groups, the sister Fellowship of AA. Every form of addictive behaviour has its own Fellowship and an equivalent 'family' Fellowship. There's AlAteen for teenagers and even, in the USA, AlAtot. It's never too early to help family members. And it's never too early to intervene in active addiction. Families can be helped to understand addictive disease and recovery. That's what saves lives.

Monica (62) loved her family to bits. They were the centre of her life. When her elder son got into trouble with drugs, she wondered what she had done wrong. She was determined to find out more. She read up everything she could. She bought a second mobile and put in an extra telephone line at home so that she could always be in touch and aware of what was going on. She gave up all her social activities so she would not be distracted or, worst of all, unavailable if something dreadful happened. Her addicted son played into this, saying she'd been a dreadful mother in not understanding the importance of feelings. By pulling the strings of her guilt, he was able to get a constant supply of money from her. And when that wasn't enough, he stole. Through constant use of drugs, his health declined. So Monica read - on the web and in newspapers - all she could learn about HIV, hepatitis B and C and even E, symptoms and signs of the use of all sorts of drugs, their appearance, the effects of overdoses, and what she could do in an emergency. She ignored her husband - who, she said, drank a bit too much for his own good but certainly wasn't an alcoholic - and her younger son to such an extent that they got fed up. I saw her ten years after those distressing times. The elder son had died of an overdose, his mother had not been able to prevent it, and she blamed herself. Her doctor put her on an antidepressant, then doubled the dose, then tried another one and then added a mood-stabiliser. He did everything he had been trained to do and as outlined in principles of best medical practice. But it didn't help Monica. She wasn't particularly disturbed by her divorce, nor by her younger son going off on his own. Her one and only concern was that, by not providing more care for her elder son, she had caused him to suffer and die. I spent an hour with her, explaining my own take on the situation. I felt that she was, perhaps, keeping her son's spirit trapped. I explained that I had had to let go of Meg's spirit. Wherever her spirit might be now, I wanted her to be free to follow her own path. That was how much I loved her. Monica never came back to see me.

Chapter 31: Training

We can change our brains as well as our bodies by regular practice.

There is a disturbing arrogance in some Twelve Step counsellors. They believe that because they have a couple of years of abstinence from one or two addictive substances – usually alcohol and recreational drugs – they think they know all they need to know in order to counsel patients.

I remember being told by my own staff, whom I had taken to Hazelden when I first established my rehab, that I could do the medical work and give the occasional lecture but not go into group.

That changed when I was invited into group therapy sessions by a subsequent treatment director. Yet even that director felt threatened when I went on training courses for EMDR, NLP and psychodrama. I was told that there should be a physical dividing line in the premises between counselling and medical work. Yet again in my life I was being told to stay in my box. I replied that I built the rehab in order to implement my own ideas and develop them.

EMDR (eye-movement desensitisation and reprocessing) is a technique of bi-lateral sensory stimulation so that the thinking brain communicates with the feeling brain. I went through the formal training provided by the staff of Dr Francine Shapiro, the American psychologist who created it. By getting patients to follow a finger moving from side to side across their field of vision, while holding in their minds an image of a traumatic event, a negative belief about self associated with that image, and emotional feelings and body sensations that also go with that event, all these distressing features can be progressively helped to become less disturbing. Eventually they are perceived merely as events. Then a positive belief, correlating with the initial negative belief is inserted as the re-processing part of the psychological process.

When I first heard about EMDR, I thought it was nuts. So I didn't attend the demonstration by Dr Shapiro herself. A year later, when I was giving a talk in a conference in Cape Cod in New England, I took the chance to see an EMDR demonstration by another member of the faculty.

I was amazed. After my training, I've been doing it ever since.

Nowadays I sit opposite the patient, with an electronic keyboard between us. The patient plays an Ab with the left middle finger and then another Ab, three octaves higher, with the right middle finger. The instruction to play the note is given by my right hand touching the back of each of the patient's hands in turn. With the head held still, the patient's eyes follow the movement of my signet ring, while talking about the particular event and its associations. In this way I put in four stimuli – sound, touch, muscular movement and eye movement – simultaneously. Also, by looking down, the patient's eyes don't get tired. In place of 24 'passes' from one side to the other and back again, I can do 400 if the need arises to keep the process going when the patient is in full flow. I find this makes EMDR much more effective and therefore quicker and less expensive financially.

I went through training in Neuro-Linguistic Programming – NLP – and hypnosis as one of a large group of students in a hotel in London. We were taught by Richard Bandler, one of the two co-creators of NLP, and Paul McKenna. They are both exceedingly skilled practitioners and hypnotists. I followed this up with small group training, first in London and then in America.

My training in psychodrama was all in America, first with Kate Hudgings in Black Earth, Wisconsin, and then with Carl Hollander in Denver, Colorado. I also attended psychodrama conferences in Washington DC. I learned how to help patients work on thoughts, feelings and behaviour while looking at their past, present and future.

I could not have been better trained in each of these therapeutic approaches. I loved being able to do something practical that helped patients to heal themselves.

I told my counselling staff that I would be glad to pay for them to have training in any therapeutic process that particularly interested them. Apart from the director of the rehab, whom I took with me to America many times, only one member of my staff took up the offer and she promptly left to work in a psychology practice somewhere else.

The end result was that I, as a full-time family practitioner doing eight four-hour consulting sessions each week in my medical practice, and also doing group sessions in the London rehab every lunchtime and evening as well as running the Kent rehab at weekends and spending all my annual holidays on training courses, finished up being better trained and more experienced than my own staff in their full-time profession.

Okay, I accept that I'm a nutter, an addict. But I'm a very happy and fulfilled nutter and addict and I could not enjoy my professional life more than I do. For that reason, I have boundless energy and I still make time here and there to do the things I enjoy, such as reading, writing and going to concerts, operas and ballets.

I wanted my counselling staff to share my enthusiasm. So, Professor Geoffrey Stephenson and I set up the first MSc training course in the UK in addiction psychology. We established this first of all in the University of Greenwich. My brief to them – in exchange for a substantial fee – was to get the university staff to train my counsellors – on day release from the rehab – in a wide range of therapeutic approaches. What they *did* was to tell my staff that, from a psychodynamic perspective, they were addicts because they had not been breast fed adequately and therefore had not formed meaningful attachments.

I took my staff – and my money – to London (South Bank) University. There my staff were taught statistics and research methods. I despaired. I resigned from the staff of the course I had helped to create.

The course is still there. It provides standard training and gives degrees that impress employers, supervisory organisations and the counsellors themselves.

But I should not be over-critical. After all, I've got my degrees already. I can't criticise others for wanting to have one. Even so, when Geoffrey offered me the opportunity to work for a PhD under his supervision, I declined. I'm not an academic. I'm a clinician. I want to learn new ideas and develop new skills.

Evie (25) told me she wanted to be a family counsellor. She felt that, as a recovering addict, she had something to offer to families in the way of telling them what they should do. I asked if she had ever seen her son on an acid trip or her daughter unconscious in an Accident and Emergency department. She was confused by my questions and pointed out that she was too young to have children likely to suffer those events. I left her to work out the inference of my questions.

Rupert (45) lasted all of one hour on my staff. He had been psychodynamically trained. I had attended the Tavistock Clinic course of lectures run by the wise and very human Dr Anton Obholzer. Subsequently I participated in a weekly psychodynamic group for six months. I felt this new counsellor might have something to offer that we lacked in terms of breadth of understanding. I took him straight into a group I was running so he could see our approach. When one of our patients was talking about her experience of early childhood sexual abuse, this idiot piped up, "Some children enjoy that". I put him on the next train to London and gave him a cheque for a month's wages. It was money very well spent.

Chapter 32: Ideas

Active addicts are robots. In recovery creativity blooms.

The Milton H Erickson Evolution of Psychotherapy Conference, established by Dr Jeffrey Zeig, is held in Anaheim, California, every four years. I sense there are two reasons for the gap:

1. To ensure that the delegates become aware that there really is progress.
2. To ensure that the 50-member faculty of the leaders in the field are not already booked up.

There are usually 70–80,000 delegates from all over the world. A few come from the UK. It is surprising any come. Why, when the NHS is clearly the best system in the world – even though it is underfunded and overmanaged – would we want to flog across the Atlantic to learn from the Americans of all people?

My irony is based on savage experience. When I built my private medical practice in 1974, a journalist from *Medical News* reported 'There seems to be no need for Dr Lefever's swanky, North-American-style practice'. Far from seeing my suggested alternative to the standard Health Centre model, which has minimal diagnostic facilities and maximal social support, she saw only that I worked in the private sector. What I hoped was to influence the NHS to copy my example. I had my own simple x-ray and ultrasound facilities, pathology laboratory, pharmacy, nursing unit and physiotherapy unit. I employed specialist staff to do the specialist work and I had a secretary but I had no receptionist and no nurse. My two part-time radiographers covered the technical side of doing ear tests, eye tests, lung function tests, allergy tests and ECGs. They also made all the appointments and, together with Meg who was a trained and experienced physiotherapist, did all the billing and dealt with the pharmacy. They all enjoyed the variety in their work. I did all the dressings, blood tests and inoculations.

We also had a few consultant specialists – a gynaecologist, an orthopaedic surgeon, an ENT specialist and a cardiologist – who came to the unit to do one session each week.

Our patients benefitted because their valuable time – that concept doesn't apply only to doctors – was respected. Their tests were done straight away and I could look at the results myself, but a visiting radiologist and a visiting pathologist gave the formal reports and maintained quality control.

The longest time patients had to wait for a specialist appointment in these most frequently needed specialities was therefore one week. Early diagnosis and treatment saves lives. Patients also shared in the happy times I and my staff enjoyed.

Over 30 years later, a socialist peer in the Department of Health, Lord Darzi, came up with the idea of 'a one-stop shop' for family practice. Ah well, give them time, give them time...

I had not proposed my unit as a model for individual practice but for group practice, with several doctors working together. I had seen units like this in my frequent visits to the USA, exploring new ideas and ways of doing things. That's why I have told this story.

I shall be exploring new ideas when I go to the Evolution of Psychotherapy Conference again this year in December. The faculty are the leaders in the field.

For Cognitive Behavioural Therapy there's Aaron Beck. He created it.

For Positive Psychology there's Martin Seligman, the head honcho.

For Mindfulness, there's Daniel Siegel, who can hold an audience spellbound for two hours on brain biochemistry.

On brain scans – with the sardonic observation that psychologists and psychiatrists are almost unique in not studying the physical organ of their particular interest – there's Daniel Amen.

Bill Glasser used to present his ideas on Choice Theory, and Albert Ellis his on Rational Emotive Behaviour Therapy, but they've both died.

Chloe Madanes will be there, talking about family therapy. Last time round she teamed up with Tony Robbins, the motivational speaker who advises presidents. There were rumblings that he's not a 'real' psychologist. Nor am I a 'real' anything nowadays. I attended a three day course in London run by Tony Robbins. Or rather, I went for the first day but didn't go back. He has a lot of communication skills but he's too far over the top even for me. "All those who agree say Aye!!"

Michael Yapko is a clinical psychologist with an interest in depression. Interestingly, he says that reality is negotiable.

Bill O'Hanlon emphasises that there are many non-medical ways of treating depression.

Christine Padesky says that changes in our beliefs should be at a gut level as well as appealing to the intellect.

Bessel van der Kolk, a psychiatrist with a particular interest in post-traumatic stress disorder, says "The body keeps the score".

David Burns says there is a revolution in motivation. He wrote a book called, *Feeling good. The new mood therapy.* I liked him but I feel good anyway.

Mary Pipher says we can revive ourselves and that all sorrow can be borne if we put it into a story.

Harriet Lerner works on transforming impossible relationships. Hmm...

Marsha Linehan works with dialectical behaviour therapy and quotes remarkable figures for the outcome of her work with addicts. Hmm again.

Donald Meichenbaum, a Canadian specialist in Cognitive Behavioural Therapy, makes it sound human.

Otto Kernberg does the same for Freudian analysis.

Claudia Black helps families through Twelve Step approaches.

John and Julie Gottman know a great deal about relationships and they appear to put that knowledge into practice.

Salvador Minuchin created Structural Family Therapy. He's almost as old as God's uncle but what a mind and what a lovely man!

Erving Polster is the main man in Gestalt.

Bob and Mary Goulding developed Redecision Therapy which combines Gestalt with Transactional Analysis...

And on and on and on, with many other magnificent speakers and practitioners, for five wonderful days.

I reckon I've got another 20 years of active professional life. That means I can get to another five of these Evolution of Psychotherapy conferences and learn more and more. Perhaps I'll learn something about treating addicts... No. I'm *sure* I shall. I'll learn a lot about lots of things. I love being in an environment where the basic currency is ideas. Lucky me.

But Americans aren't the only people with ideas even though they're thirty years ahead of us in the world of addiction treatment.

Peter McCann and his wife Margaret-Ann created the Clouds House rehab in Wiltshire before I created my rehab in Kent. Ian Wilson created Broadreach in Plymouth before that. Jim and Joyce Ditzler created Broadway Lodge, the first Twelve Step rehab in the UK, in Weston-super-Mare. It's still there. Others have come and gone. Farm Place, created by the Ditzlers in Oxshot in Surrey after they left Broadway Lodge, was a perfect finishing school. Eton, Oxford and Farm Place prepared their pupils for a well-rounded life, privileged but tough.

Peter and Margaret-Ann now run Castle Craig in Peebles, a simply lovely part of Scotland. They also have a rehab in a castle in Northern Ireland and an outpatient set-up in London. Their booklet describing their clinical research projects is the best I've seen anywhere. I'm glad to share ideas with them any day.

Charles (65) is not a nice man. He used to be a consultant psychiatrist in a London teaching hospital. He was an inveterate prescriber. He made a deliberate point of attacking Twelve Step ideas. I wonder why he felt they were such a threat.

Chapter 33: Alternatives

Try another way but make sure it works.

Psychiatrists (doctors who can prescribe drugs) and psychologists (thinkers who want to help people to live happier lives in a healthy society) tend to be at war with each other.

They fight each other over the classification of diseases. In the American Psychiatric Association, illnesses such as 'School Avoidance Phobia' – truancy in my language – are included in, or excluded from, these formal disease classifications. The medical insurance companies (on the advice of guess who) then agree to reimburse the fees of consultants treating the formally accepted conditions. Then the pharmaceutical companies find a drug to treat them.

This all came to a head in America when psychiatrists persuaded the insurance companies *not* to cover psychological treatments for addiction. Many rehabs closed. Some survived by saying their patients had 'dual diagnosis' – depression and addiction – and they put patients on antidepressants to prove their point.

I see depression – the sense of inexplicable inner emptiness – and addiction as the same thing, before and after the discovery of mood-altering substances and processes that 'work' in changing the mood. The end result of this is that psychiatrists and psychologists are *both* at war with Twelve Step people like me.

I'm not at war with them. Professor Oscar D'Agnone, a consultant psychiatrist is – at my request – my clinical supervisor. We met almost 30 years ago when we were both speaking at an addiction conference in Tel Aviv. We've remained friends and colleagues ever since.

Professor Geoffrey Stephenson, a front-rank psychologist, was right beside me for all the 23 years of my inpatient rehabs in Kent and London.

All three of us had traditional training in our respective disciplines and were registered with standard professional bodies. There was nothing 'alternative' about us.

But I tend to be seen by other doctors as a bit odd, a maverick, even not quite sane.

Early on in my career as a family doctor I supported the formation of the College of General Practitioners. The founding members, headed by Dr Fraser Rose and Dr John Hunt, wanted family practice to be seen as a serious clinical discipline with its own training programmes. They were supported by Dr William Pickles, Dr Marshall Marinker, Dr David Metcalfe, Dr John Fry and other distinguished clinicians who had happened to choose family practice for their professional career.

John Hunt was a qualified physician and surgeon, not simply at the basic level of all doctors like me but at the level of hospital consultant specialists. It would have been difficult for other doctors to cast him as a maverick, particularly when the College became the Royal College, with the Duke of Edinburgh as its Patron, and when John became Lord Hunt of Fawley. He was very much a member of the Establishment.

I have never been that and I don't want to be seen in that light. I like being on the fringe. I'm free to look at any idea, and challenge any orthodoxy, from that vantage point.

I was once offered the opportunity to be considered for a post as a Professor of General Practice in a London Teaching Hospital. But I'm not a professor. I like spending my time with patients, not sitting on committees and doing epidemiological studies. I have every admiration for doctors who have those corporate and clinical skills but it's not me.

As one of a group of trainers, with a younger doctor learning the craft of family practice at my elbow, I once commented that I did not believe that counselling skills can be taught in formal courses. Like other practical skills, they are largely innate. I was told by my peers, two weeks later, that they were glad that I had not been able to attend the previous meeting because they had discussed me and considered that I needed psychiatric help. Ha! For disagreeing with one of their basic tenets, they would have sent me to a mental institution. Later on, when I was in one, I reflected on that experience. My world seems sane enough to me but not to others. Perhaps all patients in those confined places would say the same.

Even later on, in my private medical practice, I invited two osteopaths to run weekly sessions in my office. I was sceptical on their clinical ideas but I liked the fact that their physical techniques could help my patients to get out of pain. All I could do, as an allopathically – orthodox – trained doctor, was to prescribe drugs. I didn't want that questionable privilege.

I was very happy to prescribe temporarily necessary pain killers but I felt there were better ways of managing chronic pain.

Similarly, I didn't like psychotropic medicines that act on the mind. As an NHS doctor, my prescribing costs were 40% of those of other family doctors in the area. That was largely because I didn't prescribe psychotropic drugs – even many years before I developed an understanding of addiction.

The pharmaceutical companies label these drugs as 'antidepressants', 'tranquillisers' and 'hypnotics' (sleeping tablets) even though our understanding of brain biochemistry is still in its absolute infancy. But those are fearful labels, disguising what is really happening: poisoning the brain with pills. I never prescribed them, other than to continue to provide – and help to reduce – medications that people were already taking. Addiction to pharmaceutical drugs is exceedingly difficult to treat. After all, they are the ultimate 'designer drugs'. I preferred to give my patients time to talk to me about their problems.

But – understandably – phrases like 'poisoning the brain with pills' did not win me too many friends among my professional colleagues. I was seen as too alternative.

And being Twelve Step oriented in my treatment of addicts also labled me – very much so – as being alternative. So be it.

Needless to say genuinely alternative (complementary) practitioners – using non-medical methods of treatment even if they happen to be doctors – have clear ideas on the causes of addiction and on its treatment through their approaches. Homeopaths, osteopaths, cranio-sacral osteopaths, chiropractors, naturopaths, nutritionists, acupuncturists and acupressurists, aromatherapists, Ayurvedic and Chinese medicine practitioners, hydrotherapists, specialists in biofeedback mechanisms, reflexologists, Reiki therapists and the rest all know precisely what to tell people about the causes of, and treatment for, addiction. When modern medical attitudes and treatments are bizarre – and often frankly dangerous – it is hardly surprising that these alternative practitioners flourish.

My recommendation to patients who ask me about alternative methods to standard approaches is to do whatever they want, provided it is non-invasive and therefore unlikely to cause direct harm.

However, the problem with going down alternative routes – and traditional allopathic routes – in the treatment of addiction is that it keeps people away from Twelve Step approaches that really *do* work. But I would say that, wouldn't I?

In this book I have explained Twelve Step ideas in great depth – doubtless to the fury of people who have fixed alternative ideas – and I have outlined my own journey from scepticism to adherence. I am always ready to look at new ideas but I'm not keen to re-visit ideas that I had, or learned about, 30 or more years ago when I know now that they *don't* work.

Of course, many people say Twelve Step ideas don't work. They tried them and relapsed. My reply is:

1. Become abstinent from *all* mood-altering substances and processes. There is no point in putting down one and picking up another.
2. Work – not merely recite – the Twelve Steps. Remember that the old-timers said 'These are the Steps we took', i.e. This is what we actually *did*.
3. Try whatever other approaches you like in order to see if any of them works for you in providing peace of mind in spite of unsolved problems, happy and mutually fulfilling relationships and spontaneity, creativity and enthusiasm.

My own open-mindedness took me to the Narcanon centre, run by Scientologists in East Grinstead. Bang! Just mentioning their name gets me pilloried, ostracised and all the rest. I did *not* say I support Scientology. I do not. I have no time for their E-meter device for diagnosis, any more than I have for a Harley Street 'alternative' practitioner I saw examining patients by candlelight or for cupping and some other very popular alternative remedies. But I have made a point of learning about them so that I know *why* I do not support them.

I remember only too well my initial rejection of Twelve Step ideas. Yet they have saved my life, enabled me to come through dreadful experiences and brought me great happiness. If other 'alternative' approaches achieve those results, I want to know about them.

Seeing Narcanon patients sweating out the fat-soluble drugs in their bodies in a sauna did not distress me a fraction as much as seeing patients receiving electro-convulsive therapy (ECT), or being made into zombies by well-intentioned prescribers of pharmaceutical drugs in traditional allopathic medical centres.

Peter (35) was addicted to sunbeds. It's probably how he got skin tumours. He thought he was countering Seasonal Affective Disorder. I think his 'depression' was the precursor of his active addiction to various mood-altering substances and processes. His tanorexia was the least of his problems. Getting dentists to give him intravenous Diazepam (Valium) for non-existent dental problems eventually resulted in him losing all his teeth. But there was worse to come: he was given electroconvulsive therapy (ECT) for his 'depression' (his sense of inner emptiness at the root of his addictive nature)... and he became addicted to the general anaesthetic used during ECT. He went back and back asking for more. That destroyed the human being I knew. He would have done better by taking almost any 'alternative' therapy.

Chapter 34: The Future

Live for today and tomorrow.

In the UK, in our present political climate, I have the sense that I can see the future and I know – from past experience – that it doesn't work.

Harold Wilson, a Labour Prime Minister, said his 'Social Contract' was between the government and all 'useful' people. But, as with many well-intentioned treatments for addiction, things did not work out as he may have intended.

By giving family doctors a 5% increase in wages and their staff a 30% increase, he destroyed my fully NHS practice. In those days we were reimbursed only 70% of the costs of our premises and staff. In our local area the consequence was that premises tended to be shabby and staff few and far between. There was one part-time member of staff – receptionist, secretary or nurse – to every three doctors and one full-time member of staff to every five. Because of the high cost of premises and staff in central London, many doctors had no staff at all. Consequently, their net incomes dwarfed ours. The Harold Wilson 'reforms' would have had little effect on them. They were catastrophic to us. We had to chose between cutting staff and beginning to take on private work, which none of us had ever done before. My two partners had young children and chose to stay in the NHS. I moved on.

Meg and I looked at the possibility of going to Canada or America. Because of my significant experience in socialised medicine, I was offered wonderful opportunities to work in Vancouver, Boston and Burlington, Vermont. But I'm a Londoner.

So I worked first of all out of two rooms at the back of my previous premises. I earned a lot more money than I'd ever earned – because I had minimal expenses. Then I built new premises and started taking on private patients over and above my full list of NHS patients. I gave my NHS patients free access to my x-ray, laboratory and other facilities because I was not prepared to provide two different standards of care. In any case, the marginal costs – of the x-ray films and the laboratory reagents – were minimal because I was already paying for the premises, equipment and staff.

But then the NHS regulations made my ideals even more problematic. The NHS deducts the private proportion of total income from the reimbursements paid for staff and premises. And I was also told that my waiting room was too small. It therefore didn't count towards reimbursements even though my patients rarely waited at all. I was doing eight hours of consultations a day in comparison with three or four at the most in other NHS practices. After four years I was spending more on my NHS patients than I was earning from them and I had totally failed to persuade the Department of Health, the British Medical Association and the Royal College of General Practitioners that my model of practice – by contrast with the standard Health Centre model – was one to be followed. So I resigned.

And all hell broke loose. My former NHS patients resented not having access to my private diagnostic facilities. Among other complaints, I had a six page letter of abuse from a solicitor. I don't know how much work he ever did for the state but he said I was trained by the state and therefore should work for the state for ever. I wonder now what he would say to all the 30 counsellors I trained in my private rehab.

What I learned – the hard way – was something politicians know very well: people develop a sense of entitlement. Socialists have always wanted that result. They believe it forces suppliers to improve their services. That didn't happen in the USSR or Cuba or Venezuela and it isn't happening – and won't happen – in the UK.

But free-market Conservative capitalists can be very insensitive to the needs of the incapable. There are people who do not have the wit – not just the intelligence or finance – to be able to look after themselves responsibly. They can't cope. Some people are born that way. And some bio-psycho-social illnesses – including addiction – lead to people becoming that way.

Politicians tend to stick to their Party perceptions. Conservatives want to control people. Socialists want to control the environment. Liberal Democrats are a coalition between people who want to control everything and those who want to control nothing.

In ideas on, and services for, addiction, Conservatives tend to want more restriction, Socialists want less and Liberal Democrats want to be everything to everybody.

NHS addiction services in the UK are dismal. Even in teaching hospitals the treatment of patients is grim. I shall not go on about this here. I would suggest that anyone who disagrees with my assessment should do as I have done: go to see them.

The repeated explanation – again and again – for this and other failures in state services is that the NHS is underfunded and overmanaged. That cannot *possibly* be true. A state healthcare and welfare system can be funded on *any budget whatever* provided that politicians define what will *not* be provided. – Which they'll never do because they won't be re-elected if they do.

The NHS is the ultimate sacred cow. The public at large believe that it cannot – must not, determinedly will not – be slaughtered. So we're stuck with it and stuck with the bottomless financial pit that goes with it.

I believe I should not be entitled to NHS services except for emergencies and to cover me if and when I become incapable of looking after myself. I don't want to take from the financial pot that is shared by people who have no other choice.

But, however much money we put into the NHS, the services will get worse overall because the ideas on its purpose have not been adequately thought through. And mental health services – and addiction services in particular (because the public generally has no sympathy for addicts) – will always remain bottom of the heap, regardless of how much lip-service is given to improving them. The success of the present government's appointment of a National Recovery Champion will depend on how 'recovery' is defined. If all it means is drug substitution and harm minimisation through needle exchange and promotion of safe sexual behaviour, I shall not be impressed. But the government will have its work cut out if it backs an abstinent philosophy. There are immense vested interests ranged against that.

The NHS itself is largely a male middle class organisation run primarily for the benefit of the male middle class. The diseases that affect them are the ones given the highest priority. Consultants in those specialities have the greatest kudos and the most generous financial merit awards. This is the reality I have known throughout my professional lifetime. It is gradually changing as more women become doctors but senior positions in hospital are still mostly a male preserve.

More money might be given to family practice but doctors will do exactly what they did when the Labour Party was last in power. They took the increase in income and the decrease in working hours but did very little to improve their clinical services to patients.

Yet patients still very much believe in the NHS. They think it's a good idea. My contention is that an idea that does not work in practice is – by definition – a bad idea. In Appendix IV I have reprinted ideas that I first put forward in 1977. I contended that it is the philosophy of the NHS – not its funding or its organisation – that is wrong. I see no reason to modify these ideas now.

But that's a very long way from believing that my ideas have any chance of being accepted and implemented. They don't. Even American Presidents, the most powerful politicians in the democratic world, have difficulty getting their ideas through the Senate and the House.

I know the limits of idealism. I've come up against them many times in my professional life, as this book testifies. I may be a dreamer but I'm also a realist. I believe in doing what works. My suggestions for a street-wise guide to coping with, and recovering from, addiction are as follows:

1. Teach children, as a priority,
    - how to make long-term relationships,
    - how to bring up their own children to be happy and creative,
    - how to make a profit in business by giving – and expecting to receive – quality goods and services.
2. Enact in Parliament, and acknowledge in the British Medical Association, that addiction is a bio-psycho-social illness.
3. Teach Twelve Step ideas in schools.
4. Get schools to adopt a policy of sending drug-using and dealing pupils to Twelve Step rehab and then taking them back into the school.
5. Give consequences to addictive behaviour that damages other people or society at large. The stick must go with the carrot.
6. Provide experience of Twelve Step rehabs to medical students and to postgraduate doctors, reminding them that addiction – directly or indirectly – is the major killer.
7. Develop a general awareness – particularly in politicians and in people who work in healthcare and welfare services – of the

sensitivity of compassionate helping but the fearful dangers of compulsive helping.

8. Ensure that all doctors and healthcare workers are totally familiar with The Registrar General's *Abstract of Statistics* on consumption of alcohol, drugs, tobacco and gambling and remember them as something to consider when they see people in medical, financial and domestic difficulty.

9. Even more significantly, they need to be made aware that the question, 'What about the children?' is best answered by taking children *out* of an addictive environment. An addictive home is a very dangerous place – physically and emotionally – for young children. They need to be separated from their addicted parents or carers until they are totally abstinent – even from Methadone and other drugs used as heroin substitutes. Those drugs are just as dangerous as the ones they are intended to replace.

10. Attach a Twelve Step addiction assessment and initial treatment centre to all Accident and Emergency departments. This would give addicts and their families the understanding and care they need. It would also free up the A and E departments to deal with other accidents and emergencies.

11. Establish Twelve Step rehabs in all prisons and get away from the dreadful idea of 're-toxifying' prisoners before discharge. Putting them back on heroin so that they don't overdose as soon as they are out of prison is a policy of despair. The Twelve Step programme gives hope.

12. Train Twelve Step counsellors to understand that active addicts, the very people they most want to help, will do their utmost to destroy them and discredit their ideas.

13. Develop a significant awareness in all medical staff that addiction of one kind or another affects one in six of the population. They will therefore have addicts in front of them at some time every day, whatever the precise nature of their work. Doctors also need to be acutely aware of the dangers of addiction to mood-altering prescription drugs.

14. Make politicians aware of the vast resources available to narcoterrorists who use money, drugs and armaments to undermine Western values. This problem is not going to go away by sitting down to have polite discussions – even in the United Nations. We need clear thinking and practical solutions in defence of our values.

15. Develop a vital sense in all the population that practical things *can* be done – as outlined here – to reduce the widespread terrible scourge of addiction in our personal environment.

Do I imagine these ideas of mine, based on extensive practical experience, will be warmly accepted and implemented? No, I don't. But, to paraphrase the intervention script introduced in Chapter 18, I shall say,

1. I love my country
2. AND
3. I'm concerned.
4. I observe
   - addiction problems are getting progressively worse,
   - our society is becoming progressively more divided against itself,
   - the solutions of today are not solving the problems of today.
5. I recommend the changes that I have outlined.
6. If they are not put into practice,
   - I shall be disappointed but not surprised,
   - I shall continue to put them forward at every opportunity,
   - I shall continue to look for new ideas,
   - I shall maintain my commitment to spontaneity, creativity and enthusiasm each and every day of my life.

Robert (80) is a lot younger than the age on his birth certificate. He achieves this state by generating new ideas and by filling his life with lovely thoughts, feelings and actions. He knows that he is an addict by nature so, each day, he does what is necessary to keep that destructive drive in remission.

Appendix I: Resources

Alcoholics Anonymous. aa.org
Narcotics Anonymous. na.org
Cocaine Anonymous. ca.org
AlAnon Family Groups al-anon.org

Hazelden Publishing, Worldwide. hazelden.org
Boyd-Powell Publications, UK. dbrecoveryresources.com
The Milton H Erickson Evolution of Psychotherapy Conference, America. evolutionofpsychotherapy.com
Dalgarno Institute, Australia.dalgarnoinstitute.org.au

TEDxWarwickSalon Video Dr Robert Lefever 'Why some of us are addicts.'

Appendix II: Dr Robert Lefever's Questionnaires

Full list of Dr Robert Lefever's Questionnaires on Depression/ Addiction/Neurotransmission Disease (see drrobertlefever.co.uk/ questionnaires)

1. Anxiety.
2. Depression.
3. Insomnia.
4. Prescription drugs.
5. Alcohol.
6. Nicotine.
7. Caffeine.
8. 'Recreational' (street) drugs.
9. Compulsive stealing.
10. Sex and love addiction (including compulsive use of pornography).
11. Gambling and risk-taking.
12. Compulsive use of computers, smartphones, the internet and social media.
13. Self-harming.
14. Obsessive Compulsive Behaviour.
15. Food bingeing.
16. Food starving.
17. Shopping and spending.
18. Workaholism (including hobbies and interests, cults and sects).
19. Exercise.
20. Relationship addiction (Dominant).
21. Relationship addiction (Submissive).
22. Compulsive helping (Dominant).
23. Compulsive helping (Submissive).

Appendix III: Original Book Reviews of Alcoholics Anonymous in the Medical Press

1. Journal of the American Medical Association, 10th April 1939

The seriousness of the psychiatric and social problems represented by addiction to alcohol is generally underestimated by those not intimately familiar with the tragedies in the families of victims or the resistance addicts offer to any effective treatment.

Many psychiatrists regard addiction to alcohol as having a more pessimistic prognosis than schizophrenia. For many years the public was beguiled into believing that short courses of enforced abstinence and catharsis in 'institutes' and 'rest homes' would do the trick, and now that the failure of such temporising has become common knowledge, a considerable number of other forms of quack treatment have sprung up.

The book under review is a curious combination of organising propaganda and religious exhortation. It is in no sense a scientific book, although it is introduced by a letter from a physician who claims to know some of the anonymous contributors who have been 'cured' of addiction to alcohol and have joined together in an organisation which would save other addicts by a kind of religious conversion. The book contains instructions as to intrigue the alcoholic addict into the acceptance of divine guidance in place of the Buchman ('Oxford') movement. The one valid thing in the book is the recognition of the seriousness of addiction to alcohol. Other than this, the book has no scientific merit of interest.

2. American Journal of Nervous Mental Disorders, September 1940.

As a youth we attended many 'experience' meetings more as an onlooker than as a participant. We never could work ourselves up into a lather and burst forth in soapy bubbly phrases about our intimate states of feeling. That was our own business rather than something to brag about to the neighbours. Neither then nor now do we lean to the autobiographical, save occasionally by allusion to point a moral or adorn a tale, as the ancient adage puts it.

This big book, i.e. big in words, is a rambling sort of camp-meeting confession of experience, told in the form of biographies of various alcoholics who had been to a certain institution and have provisionally recovered, chiefly under the influence of the 'big brothers get together' spirit. Of the meaning of alcoholism there is hardly a word. It is all on the surface material.

Inasmuch as the alcoholic, speaking generally, lives a wish-fulfilling infantile regression to the omnipotency delusional state, perhaps he is best handled for the time being at least by regressive mass psychological methods in which, as is realised, religious fervour belong, hence the religious trend of the book. Billy Sunday and similar orators had their successes but we think the methods of Forel and Bleuler infinitely superior.

Appendix IV: From the Literature of Helpers Anonymous

Helping others

In Helpers Anonymous we learn through the Twelve Steps how to be genuinely helpful to others and avoid being compulsive helpers. We learn how to care and not care-take.

To help other people is a lovely thing. To be kind and considerate, supportive and generous, is beautiful.

These are the building bricks of a good life. In giving to others, we ourselves receive the gifts of happiness and contentment.

Yet this very process, the basis of honest and loving relationships, is corrupted by addictive disease. The more we give, the more the addict takes and demands. And then we feel we should give even more. Each of us, the addict and the helper, is hooked into the other's compulsive behaviour in a dreadful dance.

In Helpers Anonymous we learn to see the difference between helping the person and aiding and abetting his or her addictive disease by our own inappropriate action or inaction. We learn to take the risk of leaving the addict to take full responsibility for the consequences of his or her own decisions and behaviour.

Throughout all the good times and bad, we respect the rights of the individual addict to make his or her own choices, regardless of how ill-advised or damaging we may perceive those choices to be. We recognise that addictive disease is not the fault of the sufferer and we continue to support or love the individual regardless of the decisions and actions taken. While we reject addictive behaviour and we hold the addict to full account for all his or her actions, we still do not reject the human being from our minds or hearts.

We learn to encourage his or her steps towards recovery, not through believing promises or by offering bribes for changes in future behaviour, but through responding to consistent and progressive change that is actually achieved. We learn to be deaf to the self-pity and blaming of addictive disease while responding positively to genuine attempts at change in thoughts, feelings and behaviour through working a Twelve Step programme of recovery. Yet at all times we continue our respect or love, even in the face of the very opposite of our own advice, belief or hope.

In Helpers Anonymous we also come to see that to be of real help to others we must first be willing to be helped ourselves by coming to understand our own addictive nature as compulsive helpers and treat this, one day at a time, through our own Twelve Step programme of recovery.

The willingness to be helped ourselves

When we first come to Helpers Anonymous, our concern is mostly for someone else. We search for new ideas on how to help the ones we love or for whom we are concerned. We want to understand new theories of addiction or of compulsive and destructive behaviour. We seek out new experts to advise us. In our desperation, we will listen to anybody, go anywhere and do almost anything.

Grabbing enthusiastically at each new 'solution', we become thrilled with the hope that at last we have found someone who 'really knows' and something that 'really works'.

But each time, when the honeymoon period wears off, we become sad and disillusioned – until the next time, until we find the next idea and the next expert. Then off we go yet again in our demanding and exhausting search.

But then even this new idea turns out to be no good and even this new expert is no wiser than the last. Certainly there are times, perhaps lasting weeks, months or even more, when things seem to be working out really well. We try to be calm, confident, hopeful and encouraging. But inside, there may still be the same old fears. 'Is he going to go back to it one day?', 'Is she in trouble again?', 'Why did he do that?', 'What is that so-called friend of hers doing now?', 'Suppose it all goes wrong again?'.

We learn from painful experience not to ask these questions out loud. But we say to ourselves that surely it's too much to ask that we shouldn't *think* these things. Anyway, surely it's our responsibility, as a family member or friend, employer or counsellor, to be concerned about these things. Isn't it?

Then at last, when we hear the stories told in Helpers Anonymous, we know one thing for certain: these people have been where we have been. They know our fears and hopes from the inside.

But the more we listen, the more we're struck by one particular feature: in Helpers Anonymous the members talk little about the addicts in their lives and they talk much about their own behaviour. They openly acknowledge that they work the Twelve Step programme of recovery for themselves, and not simply because they want to understand it for someone else.

Reflecting on our own behaviour, many of us recognise two things:

1. We have been care-taking for other people, wanting them to need us, for as long as we can remember, certainly for longer than we have been trying to help the particular person who brought us to Helpers Anonymous.
2. We may have neglected other people, and other responsibilities, and we have damaged ourselves and the quality of our own lives.

These two characteristics – care-taking and self-denial – have been dominant features of our lives and, in truth, they have not helped in the way we wished and they have certainly led to a lot of damage in our own lives.

At first we may be angry at having the spotlight turned on our own behaviour – just as any addict reacts in exactly this way. In time, we come to ask ourselves, 'Did my hive of activity really work?'.

Conversely, 'Was it really true, as I thought, that I didn't try hard enough?', 'Wasn't there always one more idea and one more expert?'.

We come to see that we have ourselves been caught up in our own addictive behaviour. Care-taking and self-denial have become progressive and destructive in just the same way and to the same extent as any other addictive process is progressive and destructive.

Here in Helpers Anonymous, just as in any other Anonymous Fellowship for any other form of addictive disease, we learn to look at our own behaviour and we gradually learn to be helped ourselves.

Appendix V: The Philosophy of the NHS is Wrong

1. If the state takes over ultimate health care responsibility from the individual, there are inevitable consequences:
   (a) Individuals come to think that they have rights, and hence can demand a service without at the same time having to recognize that the service is inevitably the product of the life and work and integrity of someone else.
   (b) Any thinker who allows himself or herself to be the property of someone else ceases to think. Doctors who allow themselves to become mere units in state provision of health care, rather than people who are responsible for their own philosophical and mental integrity, are not worth asking the time of day let alone their opinions on clinical or personal problems.
   (c) People often assume that the state will care for the less fortunate. When presented with evidence that it does not always do so, they complain that it should always do so - but do not feel obliged to take any positive helpful action themselves.

Thus the state is the cause of the Inverse Care Law, whereby those most in need of help may be least likely to get it. The state creates a cruel, arid, uncaring society that smothers individual compassion and human charity.

The state cannot be relied upon to produce responsible clinical care at the time that it is needed.

A true sense of commitment can only ever be the product of an individual mind and personal philosophy (even within a healthcare and welfare organisation or a business enterprise). It can never be instilled by rules, regulations and committees.

2. If resources are distributed according to need:
   (a) People compete with each other to establish their need rather than their capacity to do well on their own account.

The individual demands his or her so called 'rights' without any thought that it is at another's expense.

147

The corporate body, answerable for its expenditure of public funds, spends its budget up to the hilt – or even overspends regardless of the needs of others – so that it can demand the same again or even more the following year.

(b) Little attention is paid to the capacity of the recipient to benefit from the resource. An absolute need may be totally unchanged even after all the resource has been devoured. Meanwhile someone else with a lesser objective need is left with no possibility of the benefit that could have been his or hers because the resource has in effect been squandered.

(c) Scientific assessment of benefit takes second place to the repetitive, mindless, arrogant hollerings of political pressure groups.

3. If services are free at the time of need:

(a) Perceived needs become relative rather than absolute. Meeting a need does not satisfy: it merely shifts attention to another need.

(b) Instead of the individual patient not being able to afford treatment, the state runs out of money so that either the individual cannot get treatment at all or, alternatively, the treatment that he or she can get is not worth having.

(c) The proponents of the system point to a few people who have been dramatically helped 'at no cost' and
  - They play on the fear or pity of their listeners – and in so doing make them into supplicant pap.
  - They disregard what is happening in general to the NHS by focusing upon a few fortunate patients in particular.

(d) The state comes in time to be thought to be indispensable and with that goes every last individual freedom.

If the ideas and principles of the NHS are wrong then the practice will inevitably fail. True compassion can only be individual.

If I choose to help you or not, that is my affair but I shall reap the consequences. I have to earn my place in a compassionate society through my actions for others.

By contrast, the state can never be compassionate. When A gives the life of B for the benefit of C, but A expects the credit for himself or herself, this is the essential prerequisite for totalitarianism.

This is why Ayn Rand, the Russian/American author of *Atlas Shrugged*, a novel in which she puts forward the principles of her philosophy of Objectivism, is right when she says that the difference between a welfare state and a totalitarian state is only a matter of time.

Appendix VI: Animated Cartoons by Robert Lefever and Sol Golden-Sato on You Tube

1. Abuse and abandonment for beginners.
Childhood can be very difficult. We come through it when we learn how to do so.

2. Addiction counselling for beginners.
Learning how to be an addiction counsellor requires skill and patience as the starting position.

3. Addictive disease for beginners.
Is addiction an illness, a stupidity, a weakness of will, a product of poor up-bringing or poor choices or what?

4. Addictive families for beginners.
Addiction runs in families and the knock-on effects cause problems even in those who are not addicts themselves.

5. Alcoholism for beginners.
Many people drink alcohol with no damaging effects. Some of us do not have the gift for that.

6. Anger and resentment for beginners.
Anger is a normal feeling and we have choice on how we express it. Resentment is a killer.

7. Behavioural addiction for beginners.
Giving up addictive substances is straightforward, even if difficult. Addictive behaviours are equally destructive and must be tackled.

8. Boundaries for beginners.
Establishing healthy boundaries is not as simple as some therapists make out. It's very difficult.

9. Codependency for beginners.
This word means so many different things that it means nothing at all.

10. Communication for beginners.
Communication is what *arrives*. We may say something perfectly clearly but, if the message didn't arrive, it wasn't communicated.

11. Control for beginners.
Control over our own non-addictive behaviour is possible. Without help, control over our addiction or over other people's behaviour is not.

12. Denial for beginners.
We cannot see what we cannot see. Therefore we may believe we don't need help.

13. Depression for beginners.
Clinical depression is a term doctors and patients use when they are determined to prescribe or use prescription drugs.

14. Drug addiction for beginners.
Any substance that changes the mood has the potential to be addictive in people with an addictive nature.

15. Eating disorders for beginners.
Bingeing, vomiting, starving and purging are different aspects of the same addiction.

16. Feelings for beginners.
Addiction suppresses all feelings except blame and self-pity. In recovery, expressing feelings has to be considerate to others.

17. Gambling for beginners.
An addiction to gambling or risk-taking may be a problem with stocks and shares and property, not just with casinos, betting shops and race courses.

18. Group therapy for beginners.
We gain insight when we see our own thoughts, feelings and actions mirrrored in those of other people.

19. Health for beginners.
Physical health is straightforward. But how about emotional, mental and spiritual health?

20. Intervention for beginners.
How do we help the ones we love to stop doing things that damage them and other people?

21. Nicotine addiction for beginners.
Cigarette smoking is the biggest killer of all. It often leads to relapse to other addictions.

22. OCD for beginners.
Obsessive compulsive behaviour is part of any addiction but sometimes it is an addictive behaviour in itself.

23. Preventing addiction for beginners.
Addiction can be prevented if we know how. But we may need to forget what we already know.

24. Real Recovery for beginners.
Why should we settle for second best in our recovery or in anything?

25. Recovery and Relapse for beginners.
Recovery is a continuing process that requires continuing work, not a state of achievement.

26. Rehab for beginners.
Some addicts die before they hit 'rock bottom'. Rehabs exist to help prevent that.

27. Relationship addiction for beginners.
Relationship addicts use other people as if they were drugs.

28. Self-esteem for beginners.
Achievements, comparisons and associations do nothing lasting for self-esteem. Reaching out to help others works.

29. Self-harm for beginners.
There are many ways of harming ourselves but some specific ways can be very damaging.

30. Serenity for beginners.
We shall not achieve serenity unless we know what we are looking for.

31. Sex and love addiction for beginners.
Using other people as if they were drugs in this way gives little reward and causes great damage.

32. Spirituality checklist for beginners.
Is our recovery what we make it out to be?

33. Stress for beginners.
External stressors cause internal stress in people who don't know the difference.

34. Suicide prevention for beginners.
Who can help? And when? And how?

35. The 'ism' of alcoholism for beginners.
The -ism names an illness (neuro-transmission disease) after one of its (inappropriate) treatments.

36. Trauma resolution for beginners.
The long-term effects of trauma can be healed.

37. Causes of addiction for beginners.
We all think we know the causes of addiction. But do we?

38. Psychiatric illness for beginners.
Addiction is the same as depression but it is often confused with other conditions such as bi-polar disorder.

39. Spiritual recovery for beginners.
Spiritual recovery is a lot more than mere abstinence from one or two addictive substances or behaviours.

40. The Twelve Step programme for beginners.
The Twelve Step programme works for any addictive behaviour – if we work it.

The 40 animated cartoons listed in Appendix VI, including those illustrated here, can be viewed on social media. Here are the links:

YouTube: https://m.youtube.com/user/DrRobertLefever

Facebook: https://m.facebook.com/DrRobertLefever

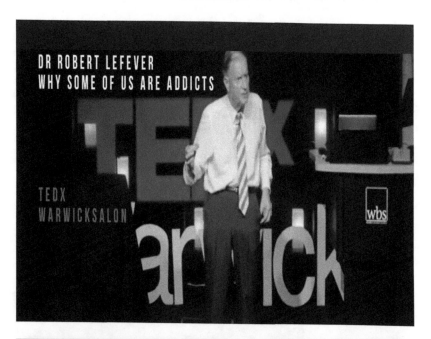

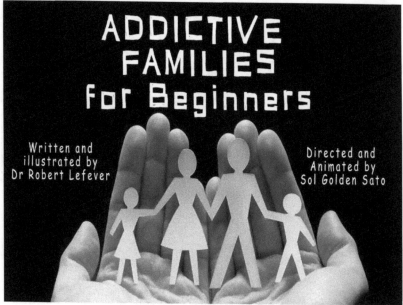

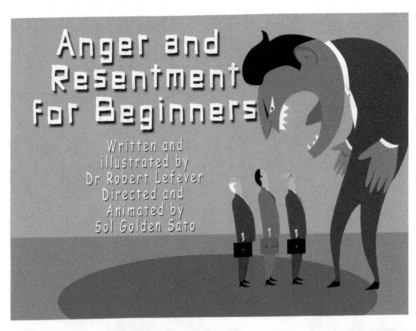

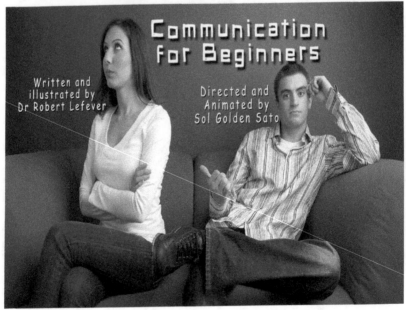

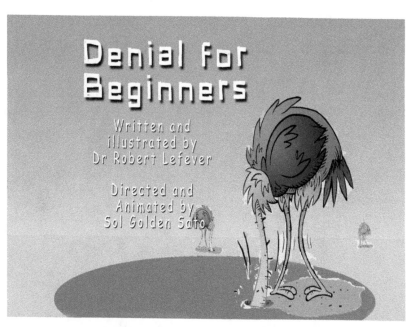

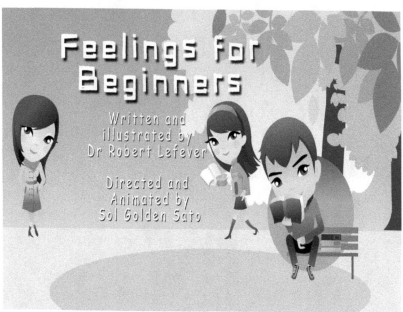

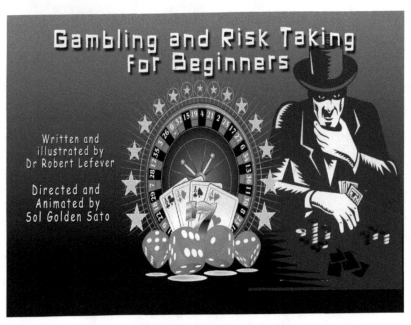

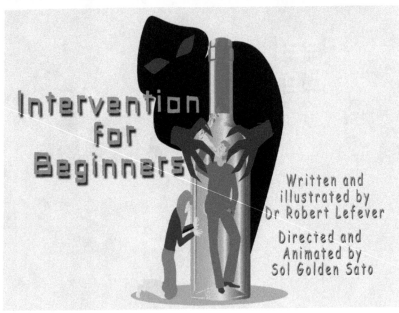

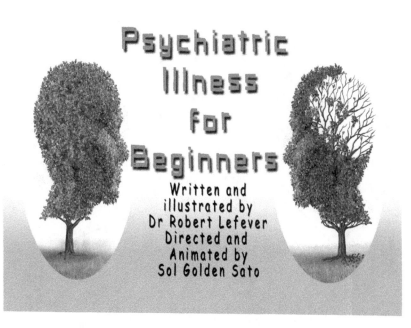

Psychiatric
Illness
for
Beginners

Written and
illustrated by
Dr Robert Lefever
Directed and
Animated by
Sol Golden Sato

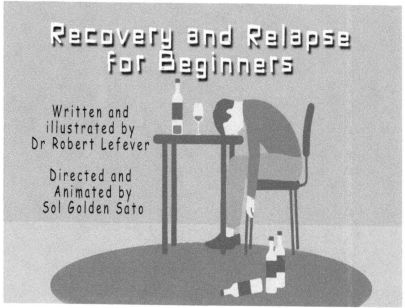

Recovery and Relapse
for Beginners

Written and
illustrated by
Dr Robert Lefever

Directed and
Animated by
Sol Golden Sato

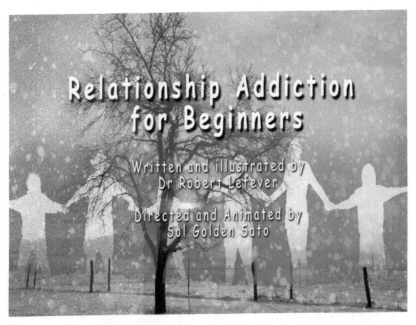

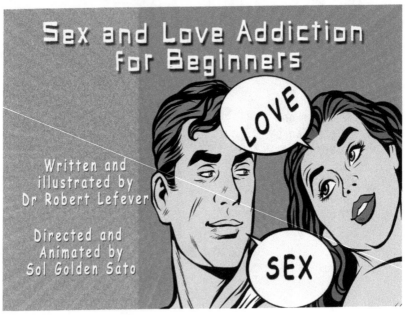

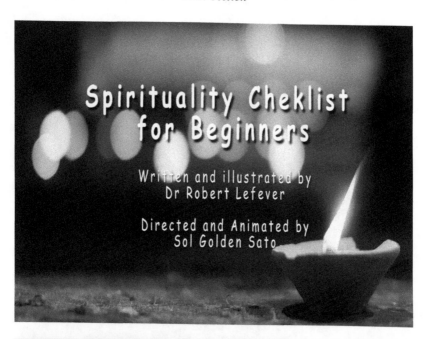

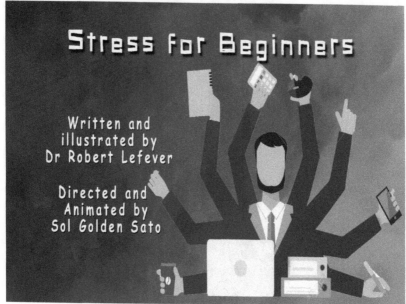

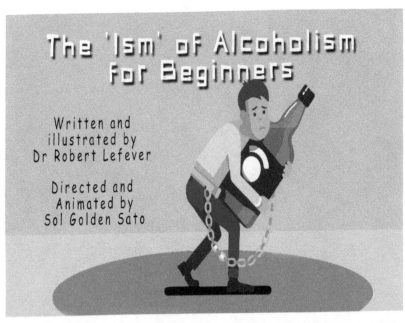

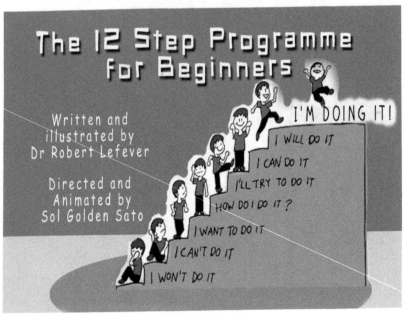

162

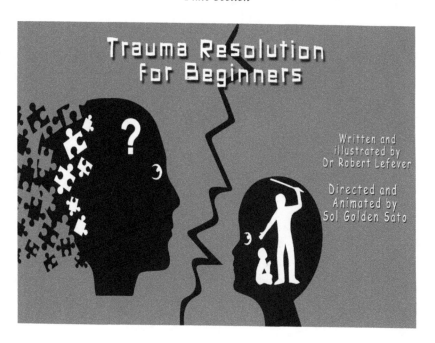

Front cover illustration:

ButterSpread © Brian Sweet courtesy of Yellow House Art Licensing.

9 781912 224487